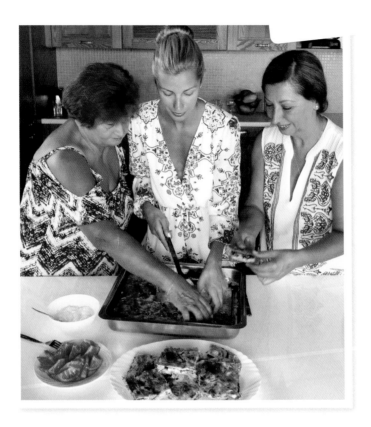

To the most important women in my life, Mom and Yiayia. Thank you for always loving me and being by my side. You have passed down your love and passion for cooking and taught me the importance of feeding loved ones with healthy, homemade meals. The hours spent learning and bonding in the kitchen are memories I will cherish forever. This cookbook is dedicated to both of you and is filled with many of our family recipes, those created out of love and laughter.

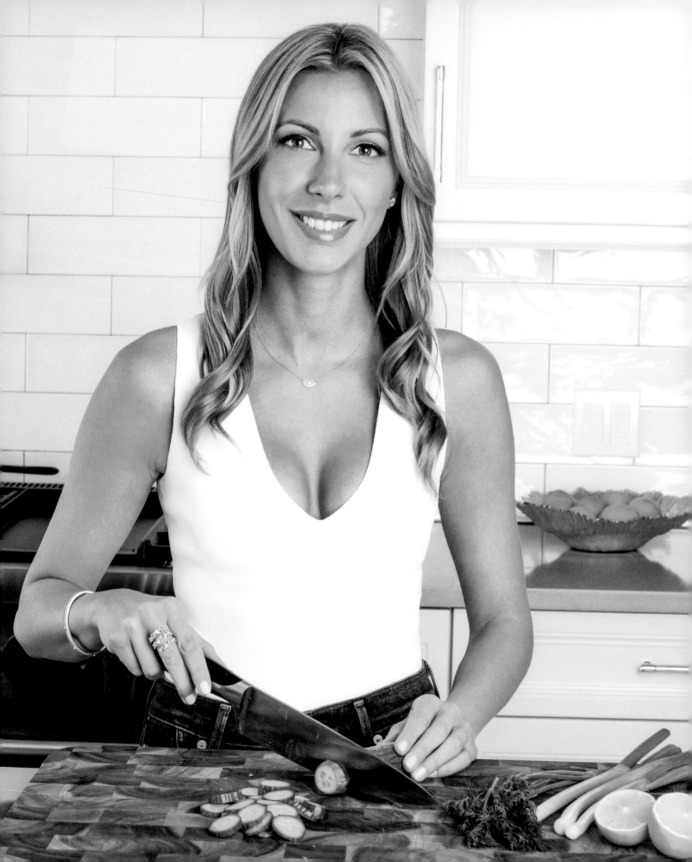

The Mediterranean Meal Plan Cookbook

Simple, Nutritious Recipes to Eat Well,
Feel Great and Look Fabulous

Neda Varbanova

Creator of **Healthy with Nedi**

PAGE STREET
PUBLISHING CO.

PAGE STREET
PUBLISHING CO.

First published in 2022 by
Page Street Publishing Co.
27 Congress Street, Suite 105
Salem, MA 01970
www.pagestreetpublishing.com

Distributed by Macmillan, sales in Canada by The Canadian Manda Group.

26   25   24   23   22   1   2   3   4   5

ISBN-13: 978-1-64567-687-4
ISBN-10: 1-64567-687-0

Library of Congress Control Number: 2022935171

Cover and book design by Molly Kate Young for Page Street Publishing Co.
Photography by Oksana Pali

Printed and bound in the United States of America

contents

Foreword

Eating real food in a processed-food world is not always easy. The temptation to eat fast food and packaged pre-made "convenience" foods is strong when these foods are everywhere—especially when you have a family and life gets busy. At times, it takes extreme dedication to cook the majority of my meals at home and save myself from pulling into a fast-food drive-through just to keep my sanity. Although I've dedicated my life to investigating the ingredients in processed food and sharing the truth with anyone who will listen, it can be hard to walk the talk all the time. I might be known as the "Food Babe" who crusades against the Big Food industry, but the reality is that I need constant inspiration to avoid processed foods and to stick to real food in my own life. This is why I enjoy listening to podcasts about how specific ingredients in our food affect our bodies. I read books daily on the health benefits of real food and how specific ingredients can prevent heart disease and cancer—and how processed ingredients like soybean oil cause damage to our bodies. I'm continuously experimenting with new recipes to motivate myself to cook at home with healthy ingredients for myself and my family. I'm always looking for like-minded people to keep me inspired and strengthen my convictions.

Neda Varbanova is one of the people I continually turn to for inspiration and motivation. She is an expert at sharing the beauty of cooking with her family, showcasing her delicious recipes with tons of vegetables and healthy ingredients. Neda's recipes are presented in such an inviting and beautiful way, so distanced from the conveniences of processed food, which makes me want to drop whatever I'm doing to make whatever she's cooking up in her kitchen. Neda embodies what the real food lifestyle is all about. She has the unique ability to inspire me to use the healthiest ingredients to cook meals that are awesomely delicious. I don't know what I'd do without people like Neda in the world to keep me on the right path.

You see, cooking and eating real food hasn't always been a part of my life. When I was a child, nearly everything I ate came from a box or a fast-food window. This eventually led me to being 30 pounds (13.6 kg) overweight—first as a teenager, then later as a professional management consultant in my twenties. I was fat, tired and stressed. It wasn't until I had a major health scare that I found the motivation to change my diet. I went on a quest to investigate all of the processed and fast foods I was eating and what I found shook me to my core. The vast majority of my "food" was composed of man-made materials from a factory. I was not eating real food. This food was DEAD—which is how I felt most of my life. I didn't have energy, I had lots of health issues, and I was on tons of prescription drugs.

I realized that I could no longer give up control of my diet to the Big Food industry. I could not continue outsourcing my health or my food, and I certainly couldn't let the food industry dictate what was healthy for me anymore. I knew I had to figure out how to make meals in my own kitchen with whole, real foods. This is when I taught myself how to cook—and everything in my life changed! All the health issues I had—asthma, eczema, allergies—disappeared. I started feeling energetic and comfortable in my own skin.

The old motto "garbage in, garbage out" is so, so true. There is no doubt about it—you feel horrible when you feed your body fast and processed food. When I began cooking, my health soared and the excess weight came off—and now, nearly 20 years later, I've never had to go on a "diet" again and have never felt better. I want everyone to feel this way! I believe that real food is medicine, and cooking has saved my life.

Cooking can save your life, too. But first, it is vitally important to make your health and wellness a number one priority in your life. You need to take a vow to yourself to shun all those processed and fast foods that bombard you at every turn, and make a dedicated effort to make cooking and eating real food a part of your daily routine. Commit to making most of your meals and snacks at home, instead of outsourcing your meals to restaurants or packaged foods. When you outsource your food, you are consuming food prepared by someone else with a list of ingredients chosen by someone else, who usually doesn't have your health in mind. When you eat food prepared by yourself, you automatically avoid hundreds of processed food additives (preservatives, flavor enhancers, thickeners, colors) that you'd otherwise be exposed to. This is the key to taking back control of your health with your diet.

Neda provides you the essential tools you need in this cookbook—along with a 30-day meal plan—to make cooking real food in the kitchen flawless and fun. Her 30-day meal plan will keep you on track so it's easier to avoid processed food temptations that try to stand in your way, because they always will.

We need more people like Neda in the world to shine a light on the beauty of getting back into our own kitchens and cooking with our families. It is my hope that Neda inspires you as much as she does me, and that you enjoy the incredible recipes in this cookbook with your loved ones. This just might save your life.

—Vani Hari
New York Times best-selling author and
founder of the Food Babe and Truvani™

Introduction

Hi! I'm Neda Varbanova, the creator of Healthy with Nedi, a platform that I made to share my love for food and wellness. I am a certified health coach with a master's in food studies from New York University (NYU) and a certificate in culinary nutrition from the Natural Gourmet Institute.

One of my true joys in life is sharing time in the kitchen with my mom and grandma cooking up delicious meals from fresh ingredients. My *yiayia* (grandma) lives in Greece, and I spend most of my summers there with her. We prepare every meal from ingredients that we pick up at the *laiki* (farmers' market) each week. This style of eating adds so much joy and vitality to my life, and it is my dream to inspire everyone to live the Mediterranean way—eating fresh, local foods, prepared with love.

I spent my childhood close to the Mediterranean, in Bulgaria, where the food philosophy is very similar. My family sat down to home-cooked meals every day. We would share our stories and connect over a table spread with vegetables, whole grains and lean meats prepared with love. My family cooked all the time and I loved observing in the kitchen. As a little girl, my mom would put me on a small stool and have me "help" by adding spaghetti to the pot or stirring something on the stove. It was a beautiful way to grow up, a dynamic I thought all families experienced. I loved eating this way, but I never realized it was healthy. It was just the way we ate in our home—no labels, just food and joy.

When we moved to the United States when I was 11, our lives and eating habits changed dramatically. I was taken aback by portion sizes and the fast-food restaurants on every corner. There were many foods I had never eaten, and I took an interest in exploring processed foods in shiny packages. This eating style began making me very sick; I would feel bloated and constipated for days at a time. I seriously struggled with my gut health and was eventually diagnosed with irritable bowel syndrome. That's when I knew I needed to return to the style of eating I had enjoyed as a child. When I began eating a Mediterranean diet again, I felt my vitality return and my digestive problems almost completely disappeared.

From that revelatory moment in high school through my master's program at NYU and in my work with clients, I have dedicated my life to sharing the pleasures of eating wholesome, fresh Mediterranean-inspired foods.

Over the years I've seen my clients experience incredible results by shifting to a Mediterranean diet. People have reported that this lifestyle makes them:

- Feel happier
- Become more energized
- Sleep better
- Experience radiant skin
- Improve digestion
- Lose weight

Experts widely consider the Mediterranean diet to be one of the healthiest ways to eat. The general principle of the diet is to eat fruits, veggies, healthy fats and whole grains on a daily basis; include weekly intake of seafood, poultry, eggs and legumes; and have moderate portions of full-fat dairy and limited intake of red meat.

For me, eating a Mediterranean diet isn't so much about eating prescribed ingredients as it is incorporating real, wholesome food and the joy and love of preparing and sharing your food into your everyday life. This lifestyle approach is centered around enjoying meals with loved ones, which shifts the focus from the food to a memorable connection. You will likely find that you will eat more slowly and engage in conversations. This allows you to tune into your satiety signals instead of quickly polishing off the food on your plate.

Don't worry, you're not going to be spending the rest of your life in the kitchen. The amazing thing about many Mediterranean recipes, and certainly the ones found in this book, is that they use minimal ingredients that are widely accessible and rarely take more than 30 minutes to prepare.

Here are the top five things that I love about the Mediterranean diet:

1. It focuses on fresh, whole ingredients.
2. The recipes are simple to create.
3. It supplies essential and nourishing nutrients.
4. It is delightful to share these recipes with your family and friends.
5. The food is absolutely delicious.

Following a Mediterranean diet meal plan may help you lose weight, and it can also support you in so many more ways that will add natural vitality to your life. Studies show that the Mediterranean diet can support cardiovascular health, has anti-aging effects, improves cognitive function and more.[1]

---

1   *Diet Review: Mediterranean Diet.* The Nutrition Source. December 2018. https://www.hsph.harvard.edu/nutritionsource/healthy-weight/diet-reviews/mediterranean-diet/

One of the other things I love about the Mediterranean diet is that you can enjoy all these benefits from anywhere in the world. Whether at my yiayia's home in Athens or back in the States, we prepare Mediterranean-inspired meals made from local and seasonal foods. More than just a regional way of eating, the Mediterranean diet can be a simple and delicious pathway to feeling your absolute best.

I grew up eating many of these recipes and have made healthy, modern tweaks to some of the classic heavier dishes my mom and yiayia used to make. This is a great way to show you that nothing is off limits. I see people who fear eating certain foods because they are "too high in carbs." Carbs are not the enemy and we need them to survive. However, if that is a concern for you, I encourage you to try simple swaps using an alternative to pasta, such as hearts of palm lasagna sheets, spaghetti squash, zucchini noodles and even zucchini ravioli if you do want to lower your carb intake. That is the beauty of food and cooking—you can eat your favorite foods by making a healthy tweak without sacrificing the taste or your waistline. Focus on making small but positive changes that will help you let go of self-criticism and allow you to feel more comfortable in your skin.

Many weight loss diet plans are restrictive and extreme, making them doable only for a short period of time. This Mediterranean meal plan provides you with a lifestyle approach to healthy eating that is a long-term solution.

I hope my recipes provide guidance and comfort and inspire you to get creative in the kitchen. You can learn to let go of deprivation, love yourself and your body unconditionally.

M. Varbanova

The 30-Day Mediterranean Meal Plan

I designed the 30-day Mediterranean meal plan and the accompanying recipes as a blueprint to guide you toward a more healthy and joyful life. With its focus on fresh, whole foods and simple-to-create menus, this meal plan is much more than a diet; it is your guide to finding sustainable vitality.

After you follow this Mediterranean meal plan, I am positive that the quality of your life will improve. You will feel happier and more energized, and you will notice improvements in your sleep, digestion and skin health.

This plan isn't about giving up foods that you love. It is about focusing on fresh and nourishing foods that will support your health and vitality. Following the meal plan can reinvigorate your happiness in the kitchen, creating a sustainable lifestyle change that will keep you feeling your best for years to come.

My commitment: In this book, I have provided 30 days' worth of Mediterranean-inspired recipes for breakfast, lunch, dinner and the occasional dessert. These recipes are designed to be both delicious and healthy, to satiate your hunger, nourish your body, share with loved ones and help you rediscover the pleasures of being in the kitchen. This style of eating is what transformed my health so many years ago and I believe that it can do the same for you.

Your commitment: To see the true results of this change in lifestyle—the increased energy, vitality and joy that come with eating fresh-cooked Mediterranean meals—you must make a commitment. This meal plan is meant to be a blueprint for a healthier life, not a rigid schedule, but it is imperative that you focus on wholesome foods throughout the meal plan. Make a promise to yourself to fully commit to the joys of fresh-prepared whole foods and skip the processed stuff, for now.

That being said, we all give into temptations sometimes. If that happens, don't beat yourself up, but select a healthier choice at your next meal. I have worked with clients who would think that just because they had truffle pizza with fries for lunch means their entire day went down the drain, and they continue to make poor choices later in the day. Instead, I tell them that we all have slips every once in awhile. One bad meal won't sabotage your goals. If you had a processed lunch, make up for it at dinner with a nutritious meal made with wholesome ingredients.

Week 1 Meal Plan

	Monday	Tuesday	Wednesday	Thursday	Friday	Saturday	Sunday
Breakfast	Easy Skillet Shakshuka (page 27)	High-Fiber "Oatmeal" with Berries (page 36)	Greek-Style Eggs with Leeks and Feta (page 23)	Low-Carb Bagels with Avocado and Sunny–Side Up Egg (page 40)	Orange Cinnamon French Toast (page 39)	Zucchini Patties with Cucumber–Yogurt Sauce (page 31)	Yiayia's Spinach Pie (page 28)
Lunch	Arugula and Avocado Salad with Strawberry Dressing (page 57) and Spinach Leek Soup (page 46)	Fettuccine with Pink Lobster Sauce (page 75)	Gluten-Free Crispy Chicken with Bruschetta-Style Salad (page 90)	Nutrient-Rich Lentil Soup (page 53) with Traditional Greek Salad (page 61)	Fresh Artichoke Dip (page 153) and Lemon Asparagus Risotto (page 119)	Spaghetti alle Vongole (page 83)	Zucchini Ravioli (page 111)
Dinner	Juicy Mediterranean Chicken with Olives and Peppers (page 89) with Low-Carb Potato–Cauliflower Mash (page 141)	Oven-Baked Eggplant with Olives, Capers and Cheese (page 115)	Mediterranean Halibut en Papillote (page 72) and Broccolini with Garlic, Lemon Zest and Feta (page 137)	Seared Scallops with Pesto and Zucchini Noodles (page 76)	Chicken Parm over Zucchini Noodles (page 93)	Spicy Greek Feta Dip (page 149) and Nutrient-Rich Lentil Soup (page 53)	Roasted Beet Salad with Goat Cheese (page 62) and Juicy Low-Carb Turkey Burgers in Lettuce Wraps (page 101)

Week 2 Meal Plan

	Monday	Tuesday	Wednesday	Thursday	Friday	Saturday	Sunday
Breakfast	Raspberry Chia Seed Pudding (page 32)	Low-Carb Bagels with Avocado and Sunny-Side Up Egg (page 40)	Greek-Style Eggs with Leeks and Feta (page 23)	Fluffy Greek Yogurt Pancakes (page 35)	Easy Skillet Shakshuka (page 27)	Spinach and Feta Cauliflower Rice Quiche (page 24)	Orange Cinnamon French Toast (page 39)
Lunch	Veggie Stuffed Zucchini Boats (page 123)	Oven Roasted Sea Bream (page 67) and Red Lentil Purée (page 142)	Hearty Minestrone Soup (page 50)	Sea Bass Lettuce Wraps (page 84)	Greek Meatballs (page 106) with Refreshing Tzatziki (page 145) and Traditional Greek Salad (page 61)	Greek Butter Beans with Spinach and Feta (page 127)	Greek Stuffed Vegetables (page 102) and Crunchy Green Salad with Honey-Mustard Dressing (page 54)
Dinner	Yiayia's Meatball Stew with Artichokes (page 49)	Hearty Minestrone Soup (page 50) and Crunchy Green Salad with Honey-Mustard Dressing (page 54)	Tender Slow-Cooked Beef in Red Wine Tomato Sauce (page 98) served over Low-Carb Potato-Cauliflower Mash (page 141)	Spaghetti Squash with Lentil Bolognese (page 112)	Shrimp Scampi Linguine (page 79)	Seared Scallops with Pesto and Zucchini Noodles (page 76)	Greek Lemon Chicken Soup (page 45)

Week 3 Meal Plan

	Monday	Tuesday	Wednesday	Thursday	Friday	Saturday	Sunday
Breakfast	Zucchini Patties with Cucumber–Yogurt Sauce (page 31)	Easy Skillet Shakshuka (page 27)	High-Fiber "Oatmeal" with Berries (page 36)	Raspberry Chia Seed Pudding (page 32)	Greek-Style Eggs with Leeks and Feta (page 23)	Yiayia's Spinach Pie (page 28)	Fluffy Greek Yogurt Pancakes (page 35)
Lunch	Spinach Leek Soup (page 46) and Creamy Baba Ganoush (page 150)	Veggie-Packed Quinoa Salad with Roast-ed Salmon (page 80)	Gluten-Free Crispy Chicken with Bruschetta Style-Salad (page 90)	Buckwheat Salad with Arugula and Feta (page 58) with Roasted Red Pepper Hummus (page 146)	Quick and Easy Shrimp Saganaki (page 71) and Grilled Zucchini with Mint and Pine Nuts (page 138)	Pork Tenderloin in Creamy Mushroom Sauce (page 94) and Baby Potatoes with Garlic and Dill (page 134)	Lemon Asparagus Risotto (page 119) and Crunchy Green Salad with Honey–Mustard Dressing (page 54)
Dinner	Low-Carb Lasagna with Mushrooms and Meat Ragu (page 97)	Red Lentil Spaghetti with Artichokes and Olives (page 128)	Hearty Minestrone Soup (page 50) and Spicy Greek Feta Dip (page 149)	Greek-Style Salmon Kebabs with Dill and Garlic (page 68)	Zucchini Ravioli (page 111)	Greek Lemon Chicken Soup (page 45)	Juicy Mediterra-nean Chicken with Olives and Peppers (page 89) with Low-Carb Potato-Cauliflower Mash (page 141)

Week 4 Meal Plan

	Monday	Tuesday	Wednesday	Thursday	Friday	Saturday	Sunday
Breakfast	Spinach and Feta Cauliflower Rice Quiche (page 24)	High-Fiber "Oatmeal" with Berries (page 36)	Fluffy Greek Yogurt Pancakes (page 35)	Raspberry Chia Seed Pudding (page 32)	Greek-Style Eggs with Leeks and Feta (page 23)	Orange Cinnamon French Toast (page 39)	Low-Carb Bagels with Avocado and Sunny-Side Up Egg (page 40)
Lunch	Roasted Beet Salad with Goat Cheese (page 62)	Spinach Leek Soup (page 46) with Arugula and Avocado Salad with Strawberry Dressing (page 57)	Creamy Chickpea Fusilli with Broccoli and Spinach (page 124)	Low-Carb Eggplant Moussaka (page 116) and Crunchy Green Salad with Honey-Mustard Dressing (page 54)	Chicken Parm over Zucchini Noodles (page 93)	Spaghetti Squash with Lentil Bolognese (page 112)	Juicy Low-Carb Turkey Burgers in Lettuce Wraps (page 101) and Broccolini with Garlic, Lemon Zest and Feta (page 137)
Dinner	Greek Spinach Rice (page 133) with Oven Roasted Sea Bream (page 67)	Greek Butter Beans with Spinach and Feta (page 127)	Herb-Crusted Roasted Rack of Lamb (page 105) with Refreshing Tzatziki (page 145)	Sea Bass Lettuce Wraps (page 84)	Yiayia's Meatball Stew with Artichokes (page 49)	Low-Carb Zucchini Roll with Vegetables and Cheese (page 120)	Greek-Style Salmon Kebabs with Dill and Garlic (page 68)

My Top Tips for Eating the Mediterranean Way

Healthy Swaps for Weight Loss

Throughout my years as a recipe developer, I have discovered many amazing foods that can take the place of heavier foods, while adding nutritional value and flavor. Below is a list of my favorite healthy alternatives that you can use as a guide for building your healthy Mediterranean pantry.

Food	Healthier Swap
All-purpose flour	Almond, coconut, cassava or buckwheat flour. These alternative flours are higher in protein, nutrients and fiber than all-purpose wheat flours.
Cow's-milk dairy products	Goat's and sheep's milk. These types of milk are the closest to mother's milk in terms of nutrient content. They also contain the A2 protein, which is usually easier to digest than cow's milk. People who develop dairy intolerances often find that sheep's-milk products are the only dairy products they can comfortably eat and digest. I often recommend purchasing sheep or goat cheese/yogurt if available in the grocery store. Most of the recipes that use dairy in this cookbook are made with goat's or sheep's milk. There are also many plant-based dairy alternatives available these days; however, these can be highly processed and contain chemicals and additives. My recommendation is to read the ingredients list and choose products that have minimal ingredients. Some of my favorite brands of plant-based dairy alternatives are Violife, Kite Hill, Monty's and Miyoko's.
Instant oats and rolled oats	Steel-cut oats, ground chia and flax seeds are excellent sources of protein, fiber and omega-3 fatty acids. They contain fewer carbohydrates and more fiber than instant or rolled oats. Although the nutritional content between steel-cut and instant oats is relatively similar, the effects on blood sugar are not. The minimally processed steel-cut oats and seeds take longer to digest, and have a lower glycemic index than rolled or instant oats. If you do choose to eat instant or rolled oats, optimize satiety and prevent blood sugar spikes by adding healthy fats, protein and fiber. You can do this by stirring in a spoonful of nut butter or tossing in some chia seeds, hemp seeds, flax seeds or slivered almonds.
Oat milk	Unsweetened almond milk or coconut milk. These alternatives are lower in calories, fat and sugar than oat milk. The sugar in oat milk is a specific type called maltose, which is unique in that it has a high glycemic index. That means it raises blood sugar more rapidly than other types of carbohydrates. There are many other plant milks besides almond or coconut, but some of them have additives and sugars. Read the labels carefully to choose products that are minimally processed when possible. Unsweetened is the best way to go.

Food	Healthier Swap
Pasta	Zucchini noodles, spaghetti squash, kelp noodles, hearts of palm noodles. Swapping out traditional pasta for vegetable-based pastas can decrease overall calorie consumption and increase vegetable consumption—a win-win. Try pastas made with brown rice, lentils, chickpeas, quinoa or whole wheat, which are available in most grocery stores.
Refined white bread	Sourdough bread. Sourdough is lower in gluten than other breads and acts as a prebiotic, which means that the fiber in the bread helps feed the "good" bacteria in your intestines. It's less likely to spike your blood sugar levels, which makes it an option for people who are monitoring their blood sugar. Other alternatives are Ezekiel Bread, which is sprouted whole grain bread. It is high in fiber, vitamins and minerals and may have less of an impact on blood sugar levels. You can also look for 100% sprouted rye bread or flax bread.
Rice	Cauliflower rice, hearts of palm rice and quinoa. Opting for ancient grains or vegetable-based alternatives can increase the nutritive value of your food.
Vegetable oil	Extra virgin olive oil (EVOO) and avocado oil. Many vegetable oils are processed and are high in omega-6 fatty acids, which can cause inflammation in high amounts. EVOO, on the other hand, supplies numerous benefits, including fighting inflammation. Avocado oil is a heart-healthy oil that is high in oleic acid, which is an unsaturated fat. It's unrefined like EVOO but it has a higher smoking point, which means it can be used to cook at higher heat.
White sugar	Honey, coconut sugar and monkfruit sweetener. An overconsumption of added sugar can lead to chronic diseases such as diabetes, obesity and heart disease.[1] Natural, less refined sugars are slightly better options than refined white sugar, though should still be consumed in moderation.

---

1   *The Sweet Danger of Sugar.* Harvard Health. January 6, 2022. https://www.health.harvard.edu/heart-health/the-sweet-danger-of-sugar

Intermittent Fasting

Although this book provides a meal plan that includes breakfast, lunch and dinner for each day, I don't want you to feel that you must follow it exactly. The most important thing is that you listen to your body. You might not be hungry the moment you wake up, and that's okay. On any given day, you can do what you feel will nourish you the most, whether it be to skip lunch or eat a heartier breakfast.

I personally fast for 14 to 16 hours per night, 3 to 4 days a week. For me, this might mean eating my last meal at 6 p.m. and then eating breakfast at 10 a.m. the next day, or finishing dinner 8 p.m. and then eating lunch at 12 p.m. the next day. I find that this type of fasting is manageable because it fits my natural hunger cycles. Researchers are beginning to find that intermittent fasting can benefit health in so many ways, such as decreasing inflammation, clearing out damaged cell parts and improving heart health.

If you want to try intermittent fasting, check with your doctor first. If you get a green light, first pay attention to when you naturally feel hungry and work from there to build your schedule. It is important to note that intermittent fasting doesn't work for everyone. Some people might have a condition that doesn't allow this type of schedule and others might simply find it so challenging that they end up in a cycle of hunger and overeating, which isn't healthy. The goal is not to feel hungry, but simply to eat nourishing, wholesome foods when your body needs them.

Fresh Juices for Glowing Skin

On mornings when I don't feel hungry, I skip breakfast and opt for a green juice instead. Drinking my vegetables gives me energy, fills my body with vitamins and keeps my skin feeling radiant. Green juice is basically vegetables stripped of fiber, which has its positives and negatives. Fiber is absolutely essential for a healthy diet, so make sure that you're eating fresh vegetables as well as drinking them in your juice. That being said, a glass of green juice can give you a burst of vitamins and minerals while letting your digestive system rest. I usually keep fruit to a bare minimum in my pressed juice because fruit without fiber is pure sugar! If you do use a bit of fruit juice for flavor, keep the portion size small.

Here are some of my favorite homemade juice combos. Each recipe makes one serving.

Sweet Greens	Power Greens	Orange Delight
1 cucumber	3 ribs celery	1 cucumber
3 pieces kale	1 cup (25 g) spinach	1 carrot
½ lemon	1 cucumber	1 orange
1-inch (2.5-cm) piece ginger	½ lemon	½ grapefruit
½ green apple	2-inch (5-cm) piece ginger	2-inch (5-cm) piece ginger
7 stems cilantro (leaves and stems)		2-inch (5-cm) piece turmeric root

Tropical Sensation

½ cup (85 g) pineapple

1 cucumber

1 cup (25 g) spinach

½ lemon

2-inch (5-cm) piece ginger

7 stems mint (leaves and stems)

Morning Greens

3 pieces kale

1 cup (35 g) romaine

½ bulb fennel

7 stems mint (leaves and stems)

½ lemon

1 cucumber

Vitamin Boost

1 cup (25 g) spinach

1 green bell pepper

7 stems parsley (leaves and stems)

1 cucumber

½ lemon

2-inch (5-cm) piece ginger

Pre-Breakfast Habits for the Body and Mind

Start each day with a glass of warm lemon water with a pinch of cayenne pepper. This will awaken your digestive system, alkalize your body and help your body detox.

Write down three things you are grateful for in a gratitude journal. By being aware of the blessings in our life, we attract more positive vibrations. Good energy can boost our feelings of happiness and dissolve feelings of anxiety. One positive thought in the morning can change our whole day.

Dessert and Sweets as Part of the Mediterranean Diet

Dessert is optional on this 30-day Mediterranean diet meal plan. I personally don't eat dessert every day and don't usually recommend consuming sweet treats daily, especially if your main goal is weight loss. I love sipping herbal teas such as fresh mint, chamomile, licorice, cinnamon or rooibos to help satisfy a sweet tooth. That being said, I don't believe in depriving yourself of the flavors that you desire as that can trigger bingeing and overeating. I believe in moderation and encourage you to allow yourself that treat when the sweet feeling strikes. Every dessert in this book is made with ingredients that contain fewer calories, carbs and sugar than most desserts, making them a healthier go-to when you are craving sweets.

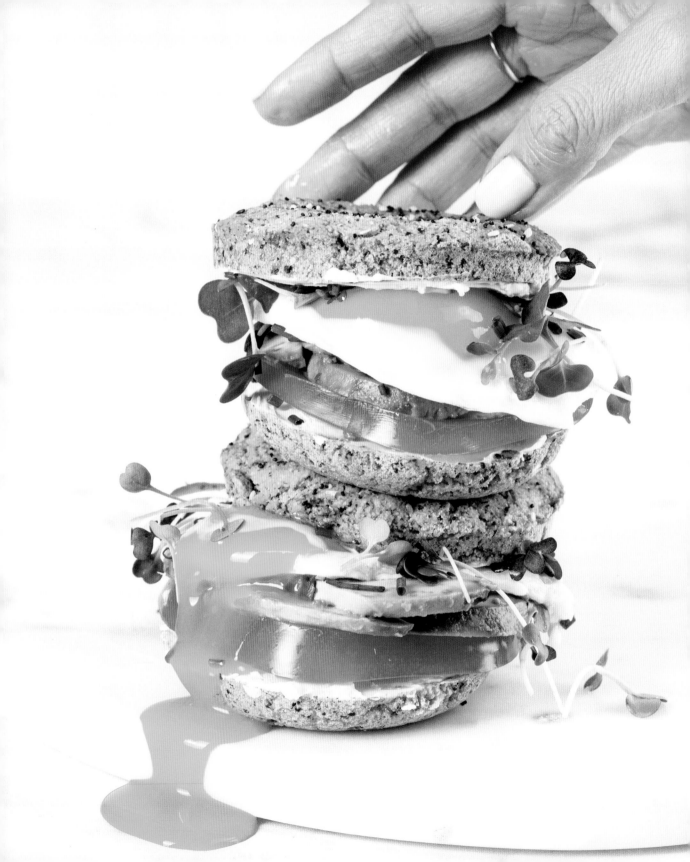

Hearty Mediterranean Breakfast Dishes

Mediterranean breakfasts remind me of joyful moments in the kitchen, shared with my mom and yiayia. Each morning, we would create delicious meal spreads made from our weekly harvest at the laiki (Greek farmers' market). Full of vegetables, eggs and fruit, a classic Mediterranean breakfast is composed of hearty and healthy ingredients that will supply you with energy for the day. I've recreated some of my favorite morning meals, like a twist on shakshuka (page 27) and a lower calorie Spinach and Feta Cauliflower Rice Quiche (page 24), to make them weight loss–friendly. I encourage you to share these dishes with your friends and family to infuse the recipes with the added benefits of love and laughter.

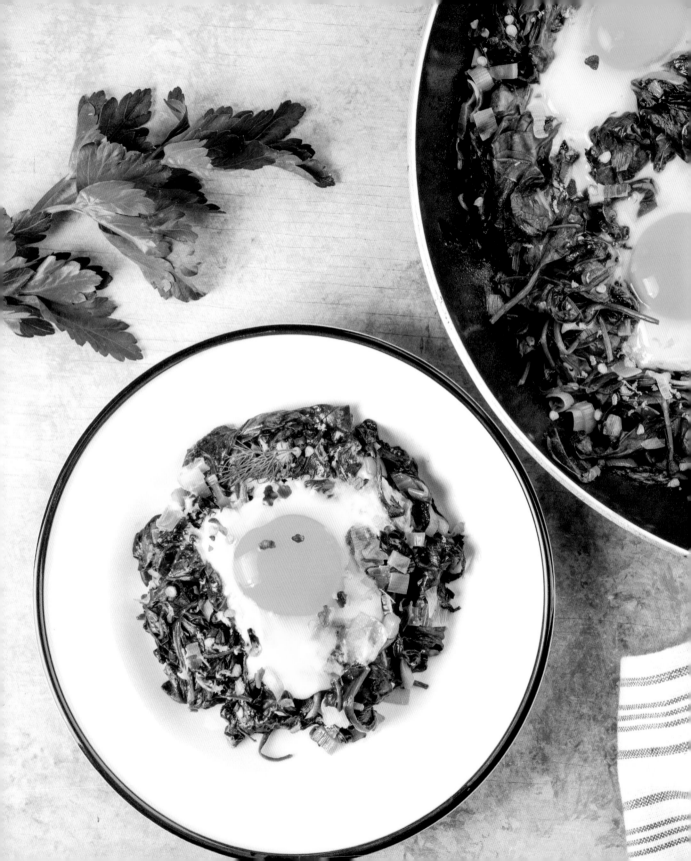

Greek-Style Eggs with Leeks and Feta

These eggs are the perfect dish for breakfast, brunch or a light dinner. There is no better taste than creamy feta with spinach and leeks. It reminds me of spanakopita, but without the extra calories or carbs. This dish is packed with antioxidants and fiber and may reduce inflammation and aid weight loss. When you cook the eggs, watch them carefully, as they are easy to overcook. Turn off the heat when the whites are firm and the yolks are tender and runny. If you prefer the eggs well done, cook them for a few extra minutes.

Makes 6 servings

3 tbsp (45 ml) extra virgin olive oil

3 leeks (white and light green parts), chopped

¼ cup (60 ml) water

1 lb (454 g) fresh baby spinach

3 tbsp (12 g) chopped fresh parsley

2 tbsp (7 g) chopped fresh dill, plus more for garnish if desired

Sea salt and pepper to taste

6 eggs

⅓ cup (50 g) crumbled feta cheese, plus more for garnish if desired

1 tsp dried oregano

¼ tsp chili flakes

Lemon zest, for garnish, optional

Heat the olive oil in a large skillet over medium heat. Add the leeks and cook for 1 minute, covered. Then add the water and continue cooking for 5 to 6 minutes, stirring occasionally, until the leeks are soft. Add the spinach, parsley and dill, and season with salt and pepper. Turn the heat to high and cook for 5 minutes, until the water starts to evaporate. Bring the heat back down to medium.

Using a large spoon, form six nests in the mixture and crack one egg into each nest. Sprinkle the feta around the eggs, then do the same with the oregano and chili flakes.

Cover the pan and cook for 3 to 5 minutes, until the egg whites are cooked but the yolks are soft. (Cook for longer if you prefer the eggs well done.) Serve hot, topped with lemon zest, feta and chopped dill.

> **Nedi's Tip:** *Frozen spinach can be used in place of the fresh spinach if needed. Thaw it in a bowl or colander and squeeze it with paper towels or your hands over a strainer to remove excess water before using in this dish.*

Spinach and Feta Cauliflower Rice Quiche

Most quiches are baked in a pie crust with eggs, cheese and vegetables. This is a healthier twist on a traditional quiche. Cauliflower rice is so versatile and can be used in many ways. It is a great way to cut down on calories and carbs without compromising the taste of a dish. It may even provide health benefits such as fighting inflammation and boosting weight loss.

Makes 6 servings

2 tbsp (30 ml) extra virgin olive oil

12 oz (340 g) leeks (white and light green parts), finely chopped

1 cup (85 g) baby portobello mushrooms, sliced

1 lb (454 g) baby spinach

4 cups (450 g) cauliflower rice

Sea salt and pepper to taste

1 tsp oregano

½ tsp chili flakes

⅓ cup (17 g) finely chopped fresh dill

⅓ cup (16 g) finely chopped chives

4 eggs

1½ cups (225 g) crumbled feta cheese

Cherry tomatoes, for garnish, optional

Plain Greek yogurt, for garnish, optional

Preheat the oven to 350°F (175°C). Line a large sheet pan with parchment paper. Lightly grease a 1.2 x 10.2–inch (3 x 26–cm) pie plate with coconut oil or olive oil cooking spray.

Heat the olive oil in a large skillet over medium-high heat and add the leeks. Cook for 2 minutes, until soft. Add the mushrooms and spinach, and continue to sauté for 3 to 4 minutes, until the spinach starts to wilt. Add the cauliflower rice, salt, pepper, oregano and chili flakes and continue cooking for 2 to 3 more minutes. Turn the heat off and add the fresh dill and chives. Stir and set aside to cool for 10 to 15 minutes until the mixture is cool enough to handle.

Once cool, transfer the mixture to a fine mesh strainer, paper towels, cheesecloth or a nut milk bag and gently squeeze to drain out the excess liquid.

In a large bowl, whisk the eggs. Add the feta and the cooled spinach mixture and stir until well combined. Pour the quiche mixture into the pie pan and spread it evenly. Bake for 25 to 30 minutes, until golden. Serve topped with cherry tomatoes and Greek yogurt.

> *Nedi's Tip: To increase the protein content, use 1 cup (180 g) of uncooked quinoa instead of the cauliflower rice. Cook the quinoa according to the package instructions then add it to the mixture in place of the cauliflower rice.*

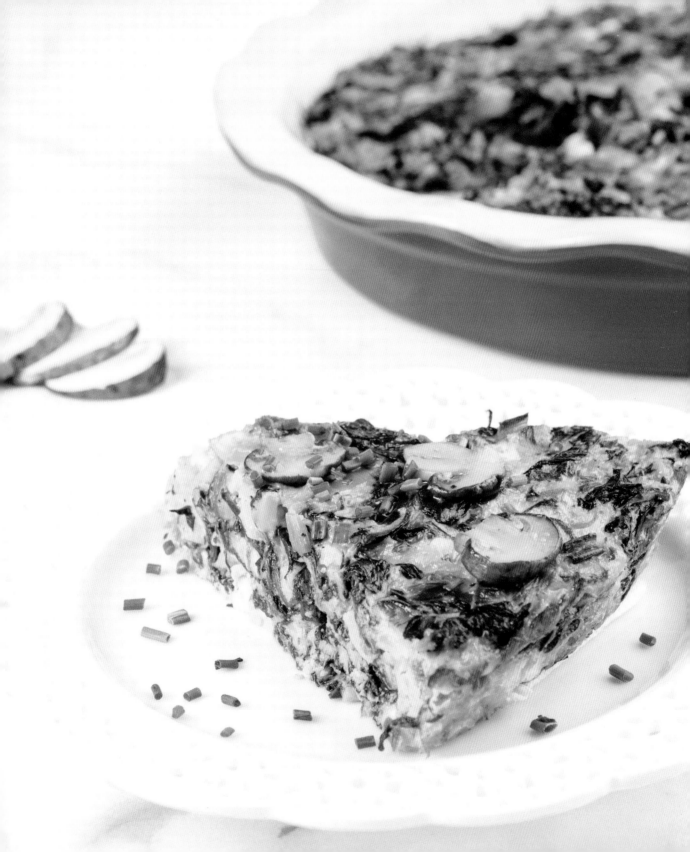

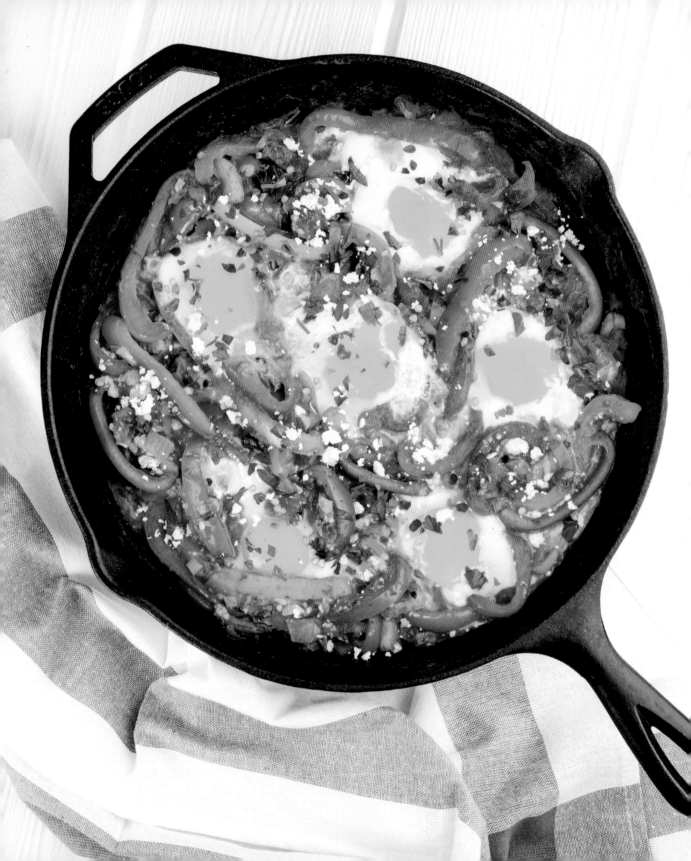

Easy Skillet Shakshuka

Shakshuka originated in North Africa and there are different versions around the Mediterranean. It literally means "a mixture" and the traditional version uses tomatoes, onions and spices as the base with eggs poached on top. There are many variations of shakshuka, and you can add different vegetables, spices, feta or goat cheese and adapt it to your taste. I like to add zucchini and green onion to make it more filling. It's a great dish for any time of the day.

Makes 6 servings

2 tbsp (30 ml) extra virgin olive oil

1 medium red onion, diced

1 green bell pepper, thinly sliced

1 orange bell pepper, thinly sliced

1 red bell pepper, thinly sliced

1 zucchini, diced

2 green onions, thinly sliced

1 tsp cumin

1 tsp oregano

½ tsp turmeric

Sea salt and pepper to taste

2 medium tomatoes, grated

⅓ cup (50 g) crumbled feta cheese

6 eggs

3 tbsp (12 g) chopped fresh parsley

Heat the olive oil in a large skillet over medium heat. Add the onion, bell peppers and zucchini to the pan. Sauté for 5 minutes, until the vegetables soften. Add the green onions, cumin, oregano, turmeric, salt and pepper. Sauté for 1 minute. Pour in the grated tomatoes (along with the juices) and simmer for 2 to 3 minutes. Add the feta and stir until mixed well.

Form six nests in the mixture using a spoon and crack one egg into each nest. Reduce the heat, cover the pan with a lid and cook for 3 to 5 minutes, until the egg whites are cooked but the yolks are soft. (Cook longer if you prefer the eggs well done.) Sprinkle with the fresh parsley and serve.

> **Nedi's Tip:** *Omit the feta to make it dairy free. To replace feta's salty punch, top the shakshuka with whole pitted Kalamata olives.*

Yiayia's Spinach Pie (Spanakopita)

If I had to choose one last meal on Earth, it would be my yiayia's spanakopita, also known as Greek spinach pie. This is the most delicious savory pastry you will ever taste—take my word for it! I grew up eating this decadent spinach pie for breakfast served with sliced tomatoes and Greek yogurt.

Makes 10 servings

¼ cup plus 3 tbsp (105 ml) extra virgin olive oil, divided

1 medium yellow onion, finely chopped

1 leek (white and light green part), finely chopped

2 green onions, finely chopped

2 tbsp (8 g) fresh spearmint, chopped

¼ cup (15 g) tightly packed fresh parsley, chopped

2 lb (907 g) spinach, finely chopped

6 eggs, divided

7 oz (200 g) plain Greek yogurt

1 tsp baking soda

2 cups (300 g) crumbled feta cheese

½ cup (1 stick/ 114 g) butter, melted

1 (1-lb [454-g]) package phyllo dough

Plain Greek yogurt, for garnish, optional

Cherry tomatoes, for garnish, optional

> **Nedi's Tips:** *I find Bulgarian feta, which is made with sheep's milk, creamier. You can find it in many grocery stores.*
>
> *The filling can be made with a mix of herbs like dill, parsley and spearmint. Some people mix Swiss chard with spinach. Have fun and get creative!*

Preheat the oven to 375°F (190°C).

Heat ¼ cup (60 ml) of the olive oil in a large skillet over medium heat. Add the onion, leek and green onions and sauté for 3 to 4 minutes, until soft. Add the spearmint, parsley and spinach. Cook until the spinach is wilted. You may have to do this in batches. If there is excess water, drain the spinach mixture and let it cool completely.

In a large mixing bowl, crack 5 of the eggs and beat with a fork. Add the yogurt and baking soda and let the mixture rest and rise for 2 minutes. Add the feta and mix. Add the cooled spinach mix to the bowl and stir until well combined.

Combine the melted butter and the remaining 3 tablespoons (45 ml) of olive oil in a small bowl. Lightly grease the bottom and sides of a 9 x 13–inch (23 x 33–cm) baking pan with this mixture using a silicone brush.

To assemble the spanakopita, lay out a sheet of phyllo dough in the pan. Lightly grease the phyllo dough sheet using a silicone brush dipped into the melted butter and oil mixture. Repeat this step twice so you have three layers of greased phyllo dough sheets.

Lay the fourth phyllo dough sheet on top of the greased layers, but without greasing this fourth layer. Top the ungreased layer with a few tablespoons of the spinach mixture. Spread the mixture evenly to cover the sheet.

Continue layering the phyllo sheets, three at a time and brushing each with the butter and oil mixture. On every fourth phyllo dough sheet, add the spinach mixture. Repeat these steps until all of the spinach mixture is used.

Lay out the remainder of the phyllo sheets; you should finish with three or four. Crack the remaining egg into the bowl with the left-over butter–oil mixture and stir. Pour the mixture over the spinach pie.

Bake the spanakopita for 30 to 35 minutes, until golden brown.

Remove the pie from the oven. Wet your hands with a little water and sprinkle drops of water over the spinach pie lightly. Cover with a kitchen towel and set aside for 10 to 15 minutes. Slice the pie into squares and enjoy while it is fresh out of the oven.

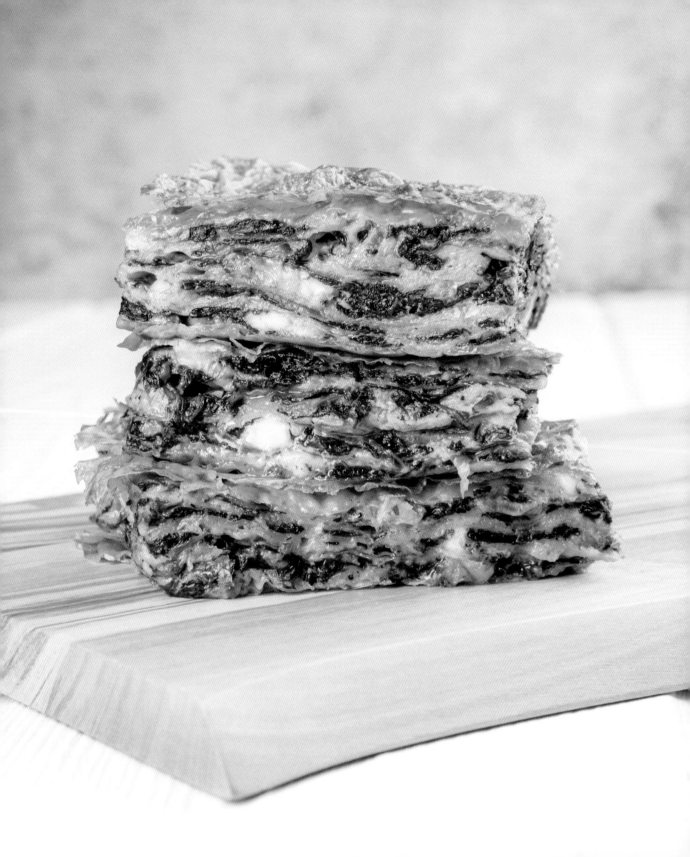

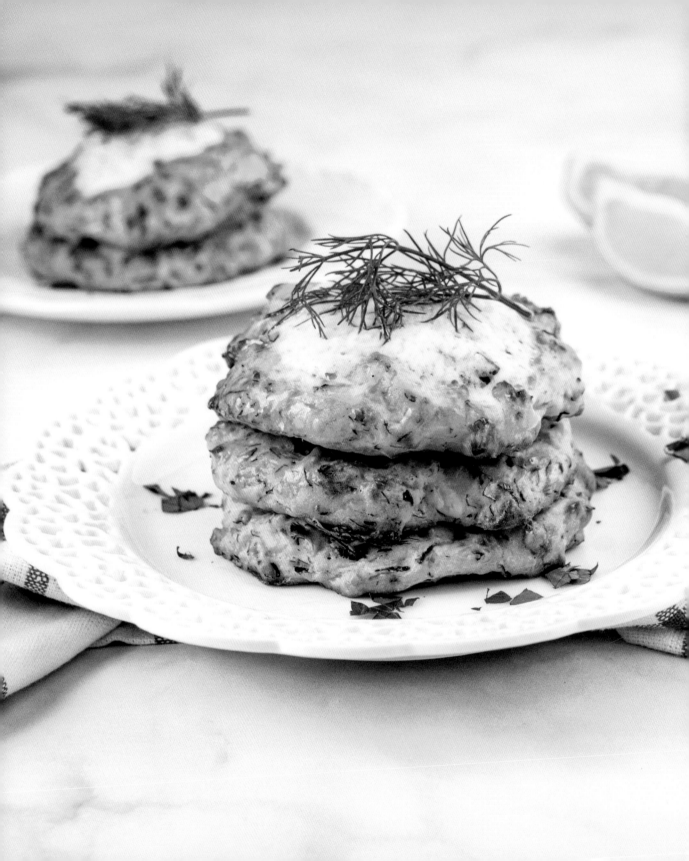

Zucchini Patties with Cucumber-Yogurt Sauce

These zucchini patties are the ultimate comfort dish. They hit the spot and it will be difficult to stop eating them! I recommend two patties per serving, along with the yogurt sauce. This is a great breakfast option, but it can also be eaten for lunch or a light dinner, paired with a gorgeous green salad and a glass of wine.

Makes 9 patties

Zucchini Patties

3 zucchini, shredded

3 tbsp (12 g) chopped fresh parsley

3 tbsp (10 g) chopped fresh dill

3 tbsp (9 g) chopped chives, plus more to serve

2 eggs

2 cloves garlic, minced

1 cup (150 g) crumbled feta cheese

1 cup (95 g) almond meal/flour

1½ tsp (3 g) dried oregano

1 tsp baking powder

1 tsp cumin

¼ tsp chili flakes

Sea salt and pepper

Cucumber–Yogurt Sauce

6 oz (170 g) plain Greek yogurt

½ cucumber, finely diced

1 clove garlic, minced

½ tsp za'atar

1 tbsp (15 ml) extra virgin olive oil

1 tsp fresh lemon juice

Sea salt to taste

Preheat the oven to 400°F (205°C). Line a baking sheet with parchment paper and set aside.

Place the shredded zucchini in a paper towel or cheesecloth and squeeze out as much of the liquid as you can.

Combine the parsley, dill, chives, eggs, garlic, feta, almond meal/flour, oregano, baking powder, cumin, chili flakes, salt and pepper in a large bowl. Mix well and add the shredded zucchini. Mix until well combined. (See Nedi's Tip.)

Form 9 patties, using about 2 tablespoons (30 ml) of the zucchini mixture per patty. Place the patties onto the prepared baking sheet and bake for 25 minutes, until golden brown.

Meanwhile, prepare the sauce. In a small bowl, combine the yogurt, cucumber, garlic, za'atar, olive oil, lemon and salt. Mix well.

Serve the zucchini patties with 1 tablespoon (15 ml) of cucumber–yogurt sauce on each patty.

Nedi's Tip: If there is excess water after the zucchini is combined with the rest of the ingredients, place the mixture back into the cheesecloth or a new paper towel and squeeze it again. Some zucchini are waterier than others and you don't want the mixture to be too moist.

Raspberry Chia Seed Pudding

The combination of sweet and tangy is incredible. This pudding capitalizes on that combo and makes for a light yet filling breakfast. Despite their tiny size, chia seeds are a nutrition powerhouse. This healthy and low-carb breakfast is loaded with fiber, protein and healthy omega-3 fats. What I love about this chia seed pudding is that it can be made ahead of time and stored in the fridge for 3 to 4 days in an airtight container.

Makes 2 servings

1 cup (125 g) raspberries, plus more for garnish

1 banana, sliced

1 tsp vanilla extract

1 tbsp (12 g) monkfruit sweetener (optional; see Nedi's Tip)

¼ cup (45 g) chia seeds

¾ cup (180 ml) almond or coconut milk

Fresh mint leaves, for garnish

Sliced almonds, for garnish

Place the raspberries and banana in a medium bowl and mash them using a fork. Add the vanilla, monkfruit sweetener, chia seeds and the nut milk. Mix well until all the ingredients are evenly combined and there are no large clumps of chia seeds.

Divide the chia seed mixture into two glasses and place in the fridge for at least 4 hours, or overnight. Serve the pudding topped with a few raspberries, mint leaves and sliced almonds.

Nedi's Tip: I find that the banana adds enough sweetness, especially if it is very ripe, but if you feel you need a little extra sweetness, add the monkfruit sweetener. You can also try this recipe with maple syrup, honey or coconut sugar.

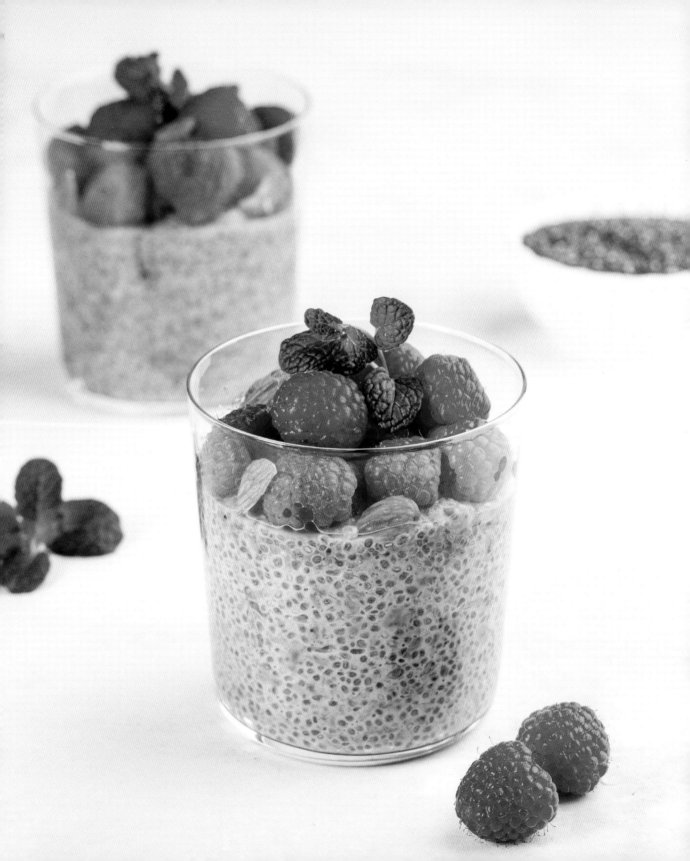

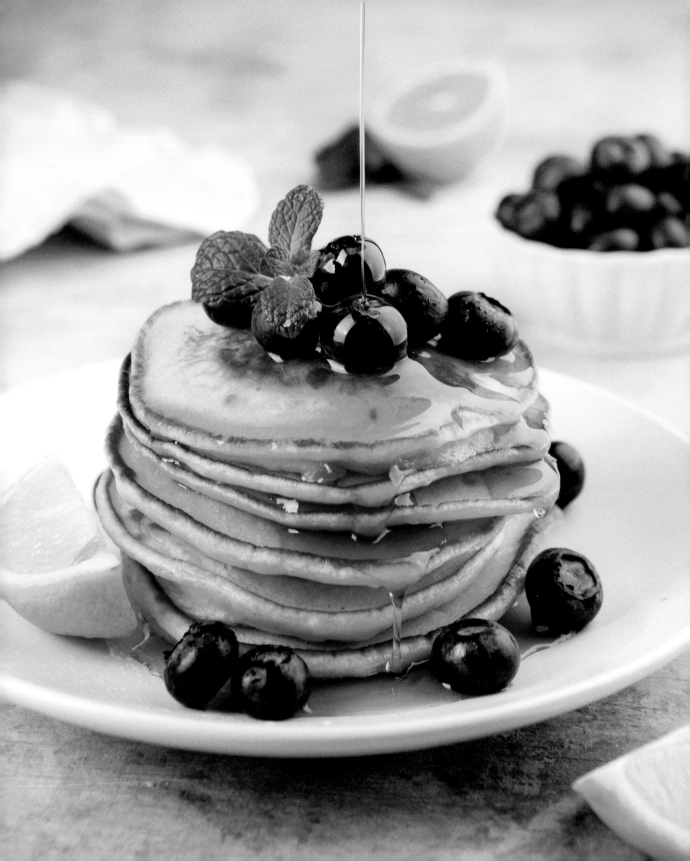

Fluffy Greek Yogurt Pancakes

Nothing is better on a weekend than a stack of freshly made pancakes. When I was younger, I loved waking up to the smell of pancakes my mom made for me. My best friend and I used to have a competition to see who could eat more pancakes and we always finished them all.

These fluffy pancakes are easy to prepare and will become a staple in your kitchen. The lemon zest adds a beautiful aroma that will freshen your senses. These gluten-free pancakes are packed with protein, which will help to keep you feeling full until lunch. Enjoy the pancakes with blueberries, maple syrup or honey.

Makes 10–12 pancakes

6.5 oz (190 ml) plain Greek yogurt

1 tsp baking powder

½ tsp baking soda

3 eggs

1 tsp lemon juice

1 tsp vanilla extract

½ tsp cinnamon

½ tsp sea salt

1 tsp lemon zest

1 tsp monkfruit sweetener or coconut sugar

1 cup (95 g) almond meal/flour

For Serving
Blueberries

Sliced lemon

Mint leaves

Maple syrup or honey

In a small bowl, combine the Greek yogurt with the baking powder and baking soda. Mix well and set aside to let it bubble and rise while you prepare the other ingredients. This step is what makes the pancakes fluffy.

In a larger bowl, whisk the eggs, then add the lemon juice, vanilla, cinnamon, sea salt, lemon zest and monkfruit sweetener. Mix well, then add the yogurt mixture to the bowl. Whisk until everything is well combined. Slowly add the almond meal/flour and whisk until mixed thoroughly.

Heat a large skillet over medium-high heat and spray with coconut oil cooking spray or coat with 1 teaspoon of coconut oil.

Using a large spoon, scoop out the pancake batter and pour into the skillet, working in batches. Three to four pancakes should fit in a large skillet. Cook them for 2 to 4 minutes on the first side, until bubbles start to form. Flip and cook for another minute. Transfer the pancakes to a plate and serve with blueberries, sliced lemon, mint leaves and maple syrup or honey.

Nedi's Tip: *Extra pancakes can be stored in the fridge for a couple of days, or frozen for up to 3 months.*

High-Fiber "Oatmeal" with Berries

This high-fiber, low-carb and 100 percent grain-free oatmeal will keep you feeling full for a long time. The unique blend of seeds and nuts mimics the texture and taste of oats. It is a much healthier option than oatmeal and it provides you with 15 grams of fiber and 20 grams of protein. The "oatmeal" is only 3 grams of net carbs and is completely sugar free. It is much more nutritious than a regular bowl of processed oats, and even more flavorful!

Makes 1 serving

2 tbsp (14 g) ground flaxseeds

2 tbsp (22 g) chia seeds

2 tbsp (16 g) sunflower seeds

2 tbsp (20 g) hemp seeds

¼ cup (60 ml) water

Pinch of sea salt

¼ tsp nutmeg

¼ tsp cinnamon

For Serving

2 tbsp (20 g) mixed berries

½ tsp bee pollen (optional; see Nedi's Tips)

1 tsp sliced almonds

1 tsp honey or maple syrup

1 tsp tahini

1 tsp fresh mint

In a blender or food processor, combine the flaxseeds, chia seeds, sunflower seeds and hemp seeds. Pulse until they are ground to flour consistency.

Heat the water in a small saucepan with a pinch of sea salt. Add the seed mixture, nutmeg and cinnamon. Stir until well combined. Add a little more water or dairy-free milk if the mixture is too thick.

Serve the oatmeal in a bowl and top with mixed berries, bee pollen, sliced almonds, honey, tahini and mint leaves.

Nedi's Tips: Bee pollen is a superfood that can be found in most health food stores. It is packed with vitamins, minerals and antioxidants. Studies have linked its health benefits to decreasing inflammation, boosting the immune system and supporting liver health. It is extremely high in vitamin B 12 and it is one of the few non–animal-based sources of this crucial vitamin.

Try this as a savory breakfast bowl with toppings such as a poached egg, sautéed mushrooms, spinach and feta!

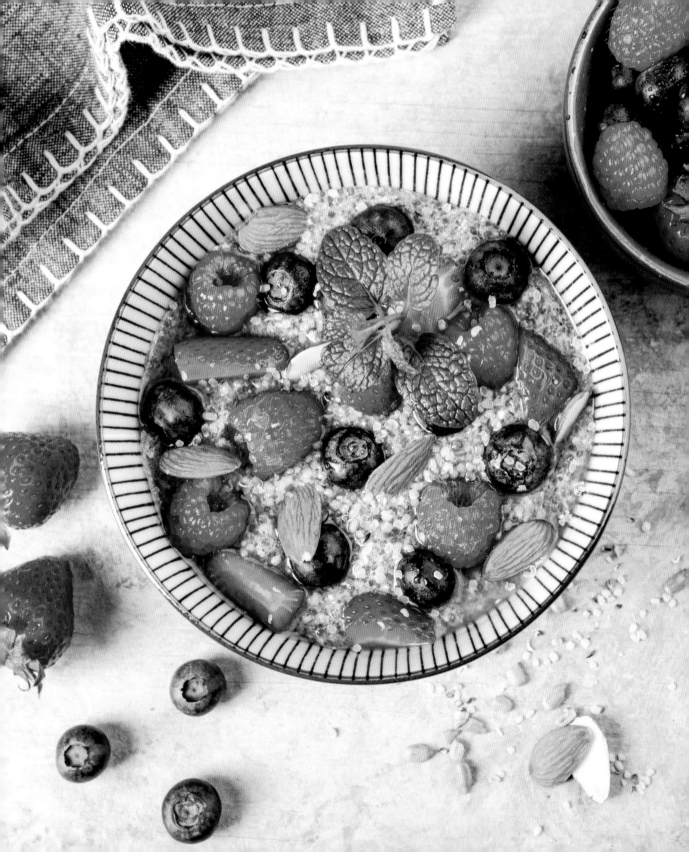

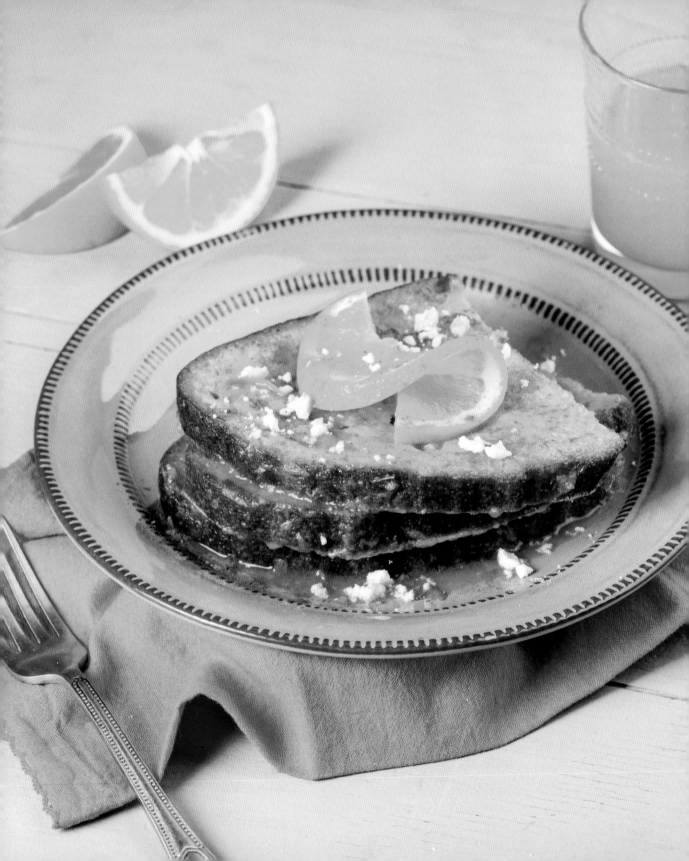

Orange Cinnamon French Toast

When I was young, I loved waking up to the yummy smell of French toast whenever my mom made it for me. The hint of orange adds an incredible flavor to this toast. I highly recommend using sourdough bread for this recipe. It is lower in gluten and easier to digest than other breads. Sourdough is made from a fermentation process and therefore acts as a prebiotic food. In other words, it is great for the gut!

Makes 6 pieces

2 tbsp (30 ml) plain Greek yogurt

½ tsp baking soda

3 eggs

Zest and juice of ½ orange

1 tsp vanilla extract

3 large slices of sourdough bread, cut in half

1 tbsp (14 g) butter

1 orange, peeled and cut into thin slices

Zest from ½ orange (optional)

Juice of 1 orange (about ½ cup [120 ml])

½ tsp cinnamon

Crumbled feta cheese, for garnish, optional

In a small bowl, mix the Greek yogurt and baking soda. Whisk with a fork and set aside for a few minutes until the yogurt becomes fluffy.

Meanwhile, in a medium-sized shallow bowl, whisk the eggs, orange juice, orange zest and vanilla. Add the Greek yogurt to the egg mixture and whisk until well combined. Dip each side of the toast in the egg mix and let them sit for 2 minutes to absorb the mixture.

Heat the butter in a large skillet over medium-high heat. Cook the toast for 3 minutes, then flip over. Cook the other side for 2 minutes, until golden. Transfer the toast to a plate.

In a small skillet, heat the peeled orange slices, orange zest (if using), orange juice and cinnamon. Bring to a boil and turn off the heat.

Serve the toast on a plate and spoon some of the orange mixture on top. Garnish with crumbled feta if you like.

> **Nedi's Tip:** *To make this recipe dairy-free, replace the Greek yogurt with coconut yogurt and use coconut oil in place of the butter.*

Low-Carb Bagels with Avocado and Sunny-Side Up Egg

These low-carb bagels are gluten-free and Paleo friendly. They are the perfect solution when you are in the mood for a bagel but don't want all the carbs. These bagels are easy to make and can be topped with any of your favorite toppings. I recommend using a donut mold to make these bagels. It really helps to create the ultimate breakfast sandwich. I love mine with dairy-free cream cheese, avocado, tomatoes and a poached egg. Another delicious option would be to add smoked salmon, sliced cucumber or feta cheese!

Makes 6 bagels

Low-Carb Bagels

1 cup (95 g) almond meal/flour

3 tbsp (21 g) coconut flour

3 tbsp (21 g) ground flaxseed

1 tsp baking soda

½ tsp sea salt

1 tbsp (15 ml) apple cider vinegar

1 tbsp (15 ml) water

5 egg whites

1 whole egg

2 tbsp (24 g) everything bagel seasoning (I like Trader Joe's Everything but the Bagel Sesame Seasoning Blend)

To Serve (per Bagel)

1 egg

2 tbsp (30 g) cream cheese

½ small avocado, sliced

½ ripe heirloom tomato, sliced

Pinch of sea salt

1 tbsp (3 g) chopped chives

2 tbsp (4 g) microgreens

A drizzle of extra virgin olive oil

Preheat the oven to 350°F (175°C). Lightly grease six donut molds with cooking spray.

To a mixing bowl, add the almond meal/flour, coconut flour, ground flaxseed, baking soda and sea salt. Mix well with a fork. Add the apple cider vinegar, water, egg whites and one whole egg. Whisk with a fork until well combined.

Spread the batter among the six donut molds. Sprinkle the bagels with the everything bagel seasoning and bake for 20 minutes, until golden. The bagels can be served right away while still warm and fresh, or allowed to cool.

To prepare the toppings, heat a nonstick skillet over medium-low heat and lightly grease with cooking spray. Crack the egg and cook for 2 to 3 minutes, until the white is firm, but the yolk is still runny. If you aren't a fan of a runny yolk and prefer the egg well done, cook for a few extra minutes. If you're serving more than one bagel at a time, you can cook as many eggs as you like in the skillet.

To serve, slice one of the bagels in half and spread the cream cheese on both sides. Add the sliced avocado on one side and the sliced tomatoes on the other side. Place the sunny side up egg over one of the sides, sprinkle both sides of the bagel with sea salt, chives, microgreens and a drizzle of olive oil.

Nedi's Tip: You can refrigerate the bagels for 5 days or store in the freezer for 3 to 4 months and reheat in a toaster or oven.

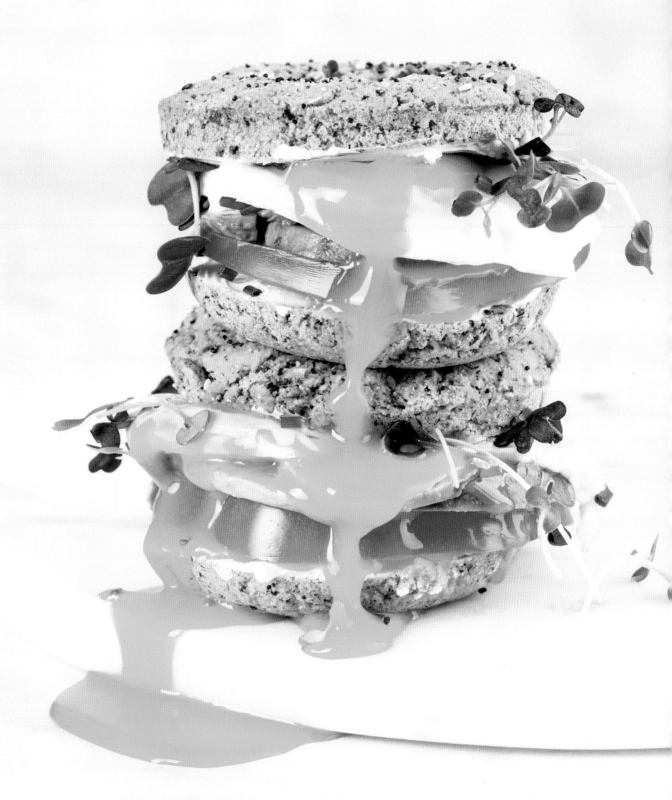

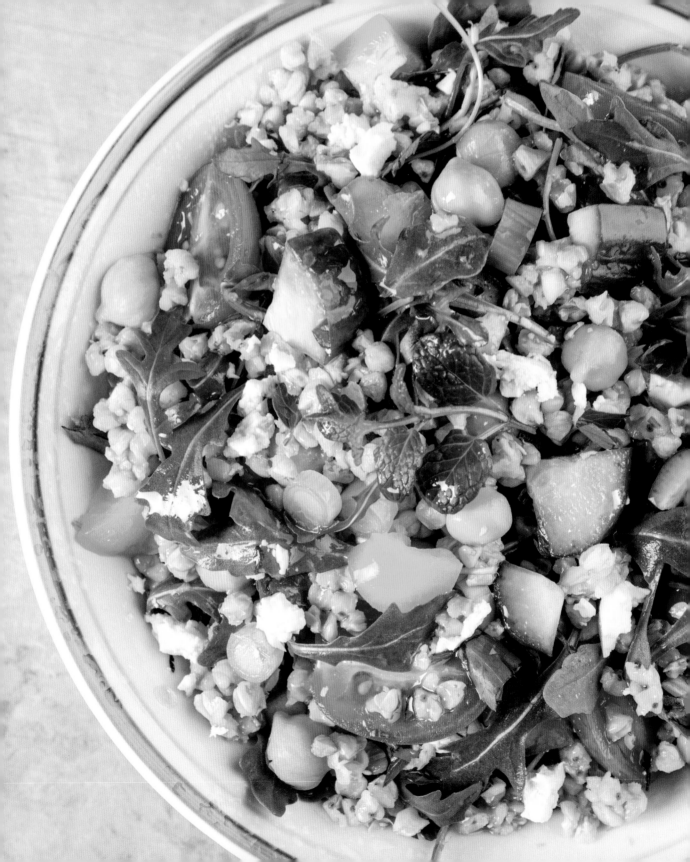

Yiayia's Starters

This chapter is devoted to soups and salads inspired by my yiayia's cooking. These dishes are designed to nourish the body and excite the appetite. Some of my first and favorite memories are of creating fresh meals in the kitchen with my yiayia. From Yiayia's Meatball Stew with Artichokes (page 49) to Traditional Greek Salad (page 61) and Greek Lemon Chicken Soup (page 45), these dishes are meant to be prepared and served with love.

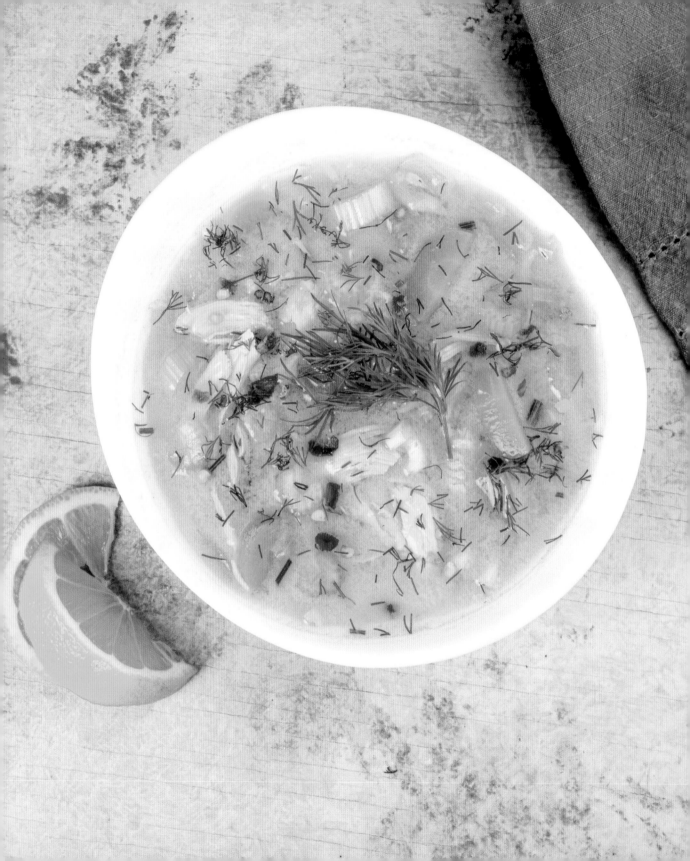

Greek Lemon Chicken Soup
(Avgolemono Soup)

This avgolemono (pronounced ahvo-lemono) soup brings back many childhood memories. My mom and yiayia used to make it to comfort me in the cold months or when I wasn't feeling well. It is one of the most comforting meals you will ever have. This recipe calls for rotisserie or leftover chicken. Using the precooked chicken saves a lot of time. The recipe is versatile and can be made with rice as listed or with orzo pasta or quinoa. Either make the soup heartier and much more filling.

Makes 8 servings

2 tbsp (30 ml) extra virgin olive oil

2 celery ribs, chopped

2 medium carrots, peeled and chopped

1 onion, finely diced

10 cups (2.4 L) chicken broth

½ cup (100 g) white basmati rice

Sea salt and pepper to taste

¼ tsp chili flakes

½ tsp turmeric

2 cooked chicken breasts, shredded (see Nedi's Tips)

2 eggs, room temperature

1 lemon, juiced

¼ cup (13 g) finely chopped fresh dill

Chili flakes, for garnish, optional

Sliced lemon, for garnish, optional

Heat the olive oil in a large pot over medium-high heat. Sauté the celery, carrots and onion for 3 to 4 minutes, until tender. Add the chicken broth, rice, salt, pepper, chili flakes and turmeric. Bring to a boil. Reduce the heat to a simmer and cook for 15 minutes.

Add the chicken to the pot and cook for another 10 minutes. Set aside for 10 minutes to cool while you prepare the avgolemono base.

To make the avgolemono base, whisk the eggs with the lemon juice in a large bowl. While whisking with one hand, slowly pour in two ladles of the chicken broth from the soup with your other hand. This step tempers the egg and allows for a silky-smooth texture in the soup. Whisk well. Steadily pour the egg mixture into the soup and stir. Stir in the fresh dill, and garnish with the chili flakes and sliced lemon if desired.

Nedi's Tips: *Typically, avgolemono soup is served with lots of fresh dill. If you are not a fan of dill, you can use fresh parsley or dried oregano.*

You can also use a store-bought rotisserie chicken for this dish. Remove the meat and shred it, discarding the skin and bones.

Spinach Leek Soup

This beautiful, rich green soup is packed with nutrients! It is full of liver-cleansing sulfur found in leeks and garlic, as well as many antioxidants and vitamins. It can be served hot or cold and tastes delicious with a little bit of crumbled feta cheese. The soup will stay fresh refrigerated for up to 5 days and it freezes well.

Makes 6 servings

3 tbsp (45 ml) extra virgin olive oil

1 small onion, finely chopped

2 leeks (white and light green parts), cut lengthwise and sliced

1 carrot, finely chopped

3 cloves garlic, minced

10 oz (283 g) baby spinach, chopped

1 ½ cups (360 ml) crushed tomatoes

6 cups (1.4 L) water

Sea salt and pepper to taste

1 cup (240 ml) plain Greek yogurt

1 large egg, room temperature

½ cup (75 g) crumbled feta cheese

2 tbsp (8 g) chopped fresh parsley

Heat the olive oil in a large pot over medium heat then add the onion. Cook for 2 minutes before adding the leeks, carrot and garlic. Cook, covered, for 5 minutes, stirring occasionally, until the vegetables begin to soften.

Add the spinach and cook for 2 minutes, stirring often, until wilted. Add the crushed tomatoes and cook for another minute. Add the water, salt and pepper, then cover. Bring to a boil and reduce to medium heat. Cook, covered, for 30 minutes.

When the soup is nearly done, mix the yogurt and egg in a medium bowl with a fork or whisk. Remove soup from the heat and let it sit for 2 to 3 minutes.

While whisking the yogurt and egg quickly with one hand, use your other hand to ladle out some of the cooled broth from the soup and very slowly pour it into the bowl with yogurt and egg. This step is crucial to get the perfect silky texture in the soup. Add one more ladle of broth the same way. When it is mixed well, add all of the yogurt mixture into the soup and stir well.

Garnish with feta and chopped parsley.

> Nedi's Tip: *If you have dairy intolerance, try using a vegan yogurt or sour cream instead of the Greek yogurt and top with a dairy-free feta cheese (or skip the cheese altogether).*

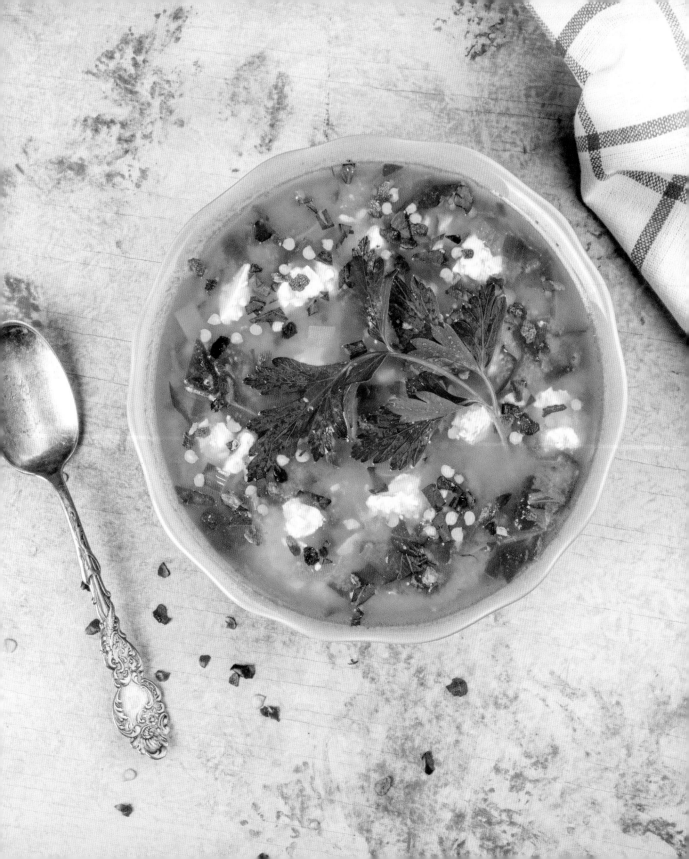

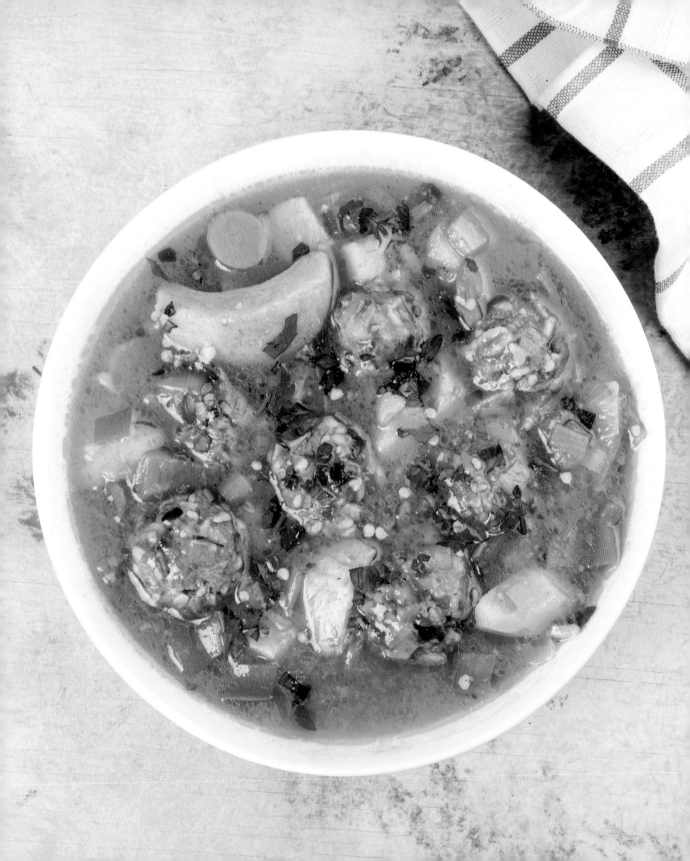

Yiayia's Meatball Stew with Artichokes

I've been dreaming about this stew since I had it last year. I had spent an entire day at the airport in Greece, trying to get on my flight back to New York City. The flight kept getting delayed and finally was canceled in the evening. I headed back to my grandma's house and she had just finished cooking this meatball stew. I was starving and it felt like the most comforting meal one could have. The next time I visited my yiayia we made the stew together and I'm so glad I got to learn her technique. Cooking together creates so many special memories for me that I know I will treasure forever. I hope you enjoy this dish as much as I do.

Makes 6 servings

2 tbsp (30 ml) extra virgin olive oil

1 leek (white and light green part), chopped

1 medium yellow onion, chopped

1 large carrot, chopped

1 red cubanelle or bell pepper, chopped

8 artichoke bottoms, cut in half (see Nedi's Tips)

1 large russet potato, peeled and chopped

2 qt (1.9 L) low sodium vegetable broth

2 cups (480 ml) hot water

1 lb 2 oz (500 g) ground beef

½ cup (90 g) dry chickpea rice or regular dry rice (see Nedi's Tips)

1 tsp cumin

1 tsp pepper

½ tsp turmeric

½ tsp cinnamon

½ tsp smoked paprika

½ tsp oregano

¼ tsp chili flakes

Sea salt to taste

½ cup (75 g) gluten-free all-purpose flour blend

3 tbsp (12 g) chopped parsley

Heat the olive oil in a large pot over medium heat and add the leek, onion, carrot and pepper. Sauté for a few minutes, until tender. Add the artichoke bottoms and potato and sauté for another 2 minutes. Pour in the vegetable broth and water.

In a large bowl, add the ground beef, chickpea rice, cumin, pepper, turmeric, cinnamon, paprika, oregano, chili flakes and salt. Mix well and form small meatballs, about 1 tablespoon (15 g) each. Spread the flour on a plate and lightly roll each meatball in the flour to prevent them from falling apart.

Gently toss the meatballs into the stew. Bring to a boil then lower the heat to medium. Cook for an hour, lightly covered. Garnish with the chopped parsley at the end and turn off the heat. Serve while hot and enjoy!

Nedi's Tips: *Artichoke bottoms can be purchased in cans from Amazon. I always have my pantry stocked with them. They are packed with fiber and nutrients and make a great low-carb substitute for potatoes. If you can't find artichoke bottoms, one or two additional russet potatoes can be used instead.*

Chickpea rice can be found from the brand Banza. I like to use it as it has more protein and fiber than regular rice.

Hearty Minestrone Soup

Vegetable soups are light, yet filling, and without too many calories. This minestrone is a classic soup that can easily be thrown together for a quick weeknight meal. You can use whatever vegetables you like or have on hand. Sometimes I like to add broccoli, cauliflower or parsnip. Try using dill or parsley instead of basil. Get creative with it and have fun. I personally like to skip the pasta that is typically used in a traditional minestrone soup; I love that the cannellini beans keep it hearty without using carb-heavy pasta.

Makes 6 servings

1 tbsp (15 ml) extra virgin olive oil

1 onion, diced

1 leek (white and light green part), sliced

4 cloves garlic, minced

1 celery rib, diced

2 carrots, diced

1 zucchini, diced

2 qt (1.89 L) water

3 oz (85 g) fresh baby spinach

8 oz (226 g) French-style green beans, trimmed and cut into 1-inch (2.5-cm) lengths

1 bay leaf

½ tsp dried thyme

½ tsp turmeric

¼ tsp chili flakes

1 large tomato, grated

Sea salt and pepper to taste

1 (13-oz [370-g]) can cannellini beans, drained and rinsed

¼ cup (10 g) chopped fresh basil

Grated pecorino Romano, for serving

Heat the olive oil in a large pot over medium heat. Add the onion, leek and garlic. Sauté for 2 minutes, until the onion is translucent. Add the celery, carrots and zucchini. Sauté for 1 minute. Add the water, stir well and bring to a boil.

Lower the heat to low and add the spinach, green beans, bay leaf, thyme, turmeric, chili flakes, grated tomato, salt and pepper. Cover the soup and cook for 20 minutes. Add the cannellini beans and cook for another 5 minutes. Turn off the heat and garnish with the fresh basil. Serve with grated pecorino Romano and enjoy.

Nedi's Tip: *This soup will keep in the fridge for 5 days or frozen for up to 6 months.*

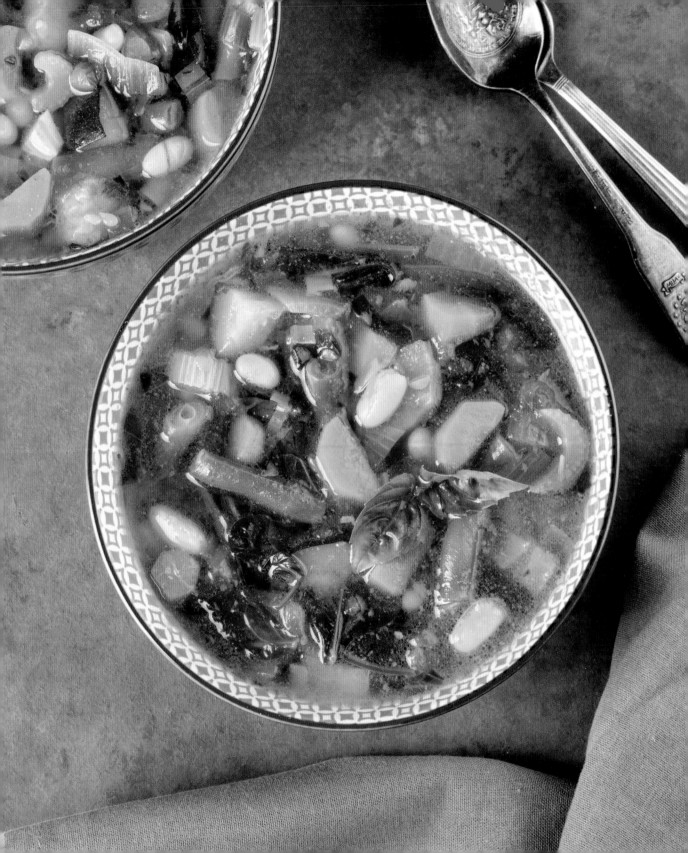

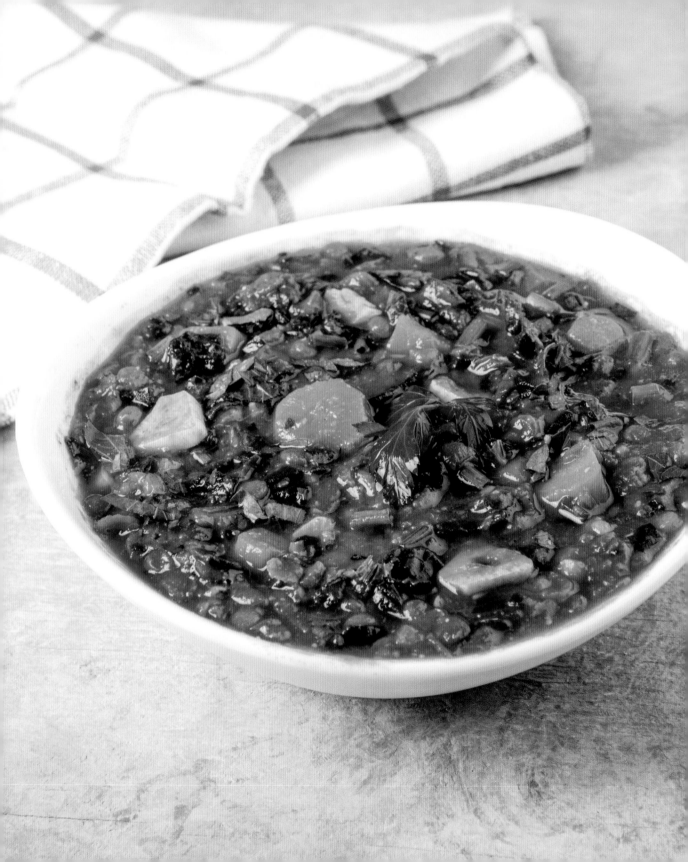

Nutrient-Rich Lentil Soup

I grew up eating this nutritious lentil soup on a weekly basis and still love to make it. There is nothing better than a homemade, comforting meal on a cold winter day. Lentils are a wonderful source of protein, fiber, iron and vitamins. The lentils in the soup can help promote digestive health, stabilize blood sugar levels, reduce blood cholesterol and increase energy. Serve the soup with a squeeze of fresh lemon juice to round out the flavors with a pop of brightness. I also love to garnish it with crumbled feta cheese but that's completely optional.

Makes 8 servings

3 tbsp (45 ml) extra virgin olive oil

1 medium yellow onion, finely chopped

2 medium carrots, finely chopped

6–8 cloves garlic, chopped

1 (14.5-oz [411-g]) can crushed tomatoes

1 lb (454 g) brown lentils, rinsed

2 qt (1.89 L) water

1 tbsp (5 g) dried oregano

1 tsp cumin

1 tsp pepper

½ tsp chili flakes

Sea salt to taste

2 cups (60 g) tightly packed fresh spinach leaves, chopped

3 tbsp (12 g) chopped fresh parsley

2 tbsp (6 g) thinly sliced chives

Lemon wedges, for garnish

Crumbled feta cheese, for garnish, optional

Heat the olive oil in a large pot over medium heat. Sauté the onion and carrots for 2 minutes, until the onion is translucent, then add the garlic. Continue sautéing for another 2 minutes, stirring occasionally.

Add the crushed tomatoes, brown lentils and water. Bring to a boil. Add the oregano, cumin, pepper, chili flakes and salt to taste. Lower the heat to medium, then cover and cook for 30 minutes until the lentils are tender.

Scoop out 2 cups (480 ml) of the lentil soup using a ladle and place in a food processor. Process the mixture until it's smooth. Place the pureed mixture back into the large pot. This step will make the soup thicker.

Add the spinach and fresh parsley, mix well until the spinach wilts, then turn off the heat. Garnish with the chives, a squeeze of fresh lemon juice and crumbled feta cheese if desired. Enjoy!

Nedi's Tip: The soup can be stored in the fridge for up to 5 days or the freezer for 6 months.

Crunchy Green Salad with Honey-Mustard Dressing

This salad is made with simple ingredients, and it has become a weekly staple in our house. I crave this salad more than anything because it is so easy to pair with any main dish. It's light, crunchy and super refreshing.

Makes 4 servings

Salad

½ head iceberg lettuce, chopped (about 4 cups [227 g])

2 cups (40 g) arugula

2 Persian cucumbers, cut in half and sliced

4 green onions, finely chopped

1 avocado, sliced

3 hearts of palm, thinly sliced

¼ cup (38 g) crumbled feta cheese

2 tbsp (7 g) finely chopped fresh dill

Dressing

1 lemon, juiced

2 tbsp (30 ml) extra virgin olive oil

1 tsp Dijon mustard

1 tsp honey or maple syrup

½ tsp sumac

Sea salt to taste

In a large bowl, combine the lettuce, arugula, cucumbers, green onions, avocado, hearts of palm, feta and dill.

In a separate small bowl, combine the lemon juice, olive oil, Dijon mustard, honey, sumac and salt. Mix well then pour the dressing over the salad. Toss a few times until well combined, then transfer to a platter to serve.

> Nedi's Tip: *Typically, when I am in Greece, I like to use valeriana greens instead of arugula. It is also known as lamb's lettuce, but I have a difficult time obtaining it in the United States. If you come across it, give it a try. It's delicious!*

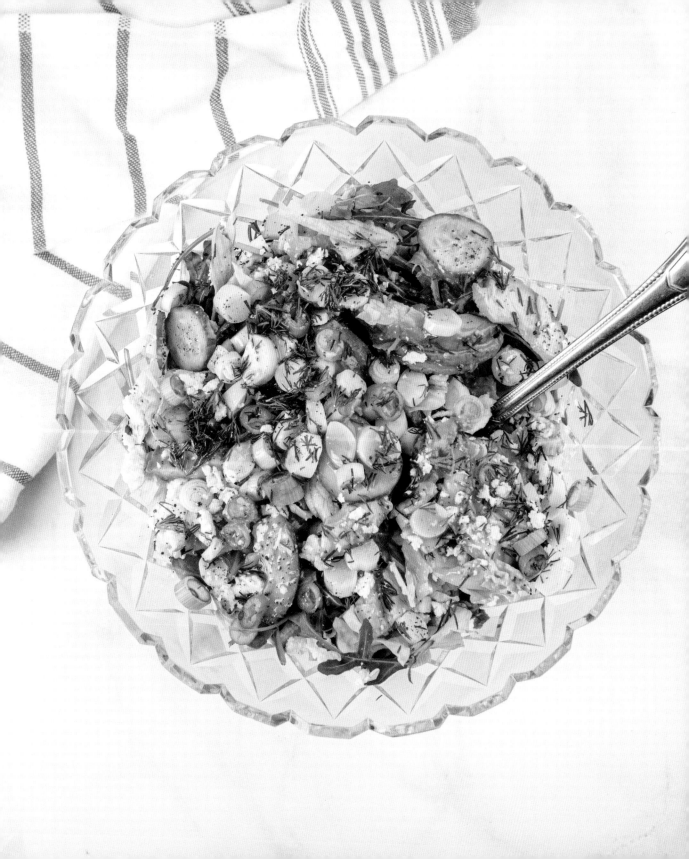

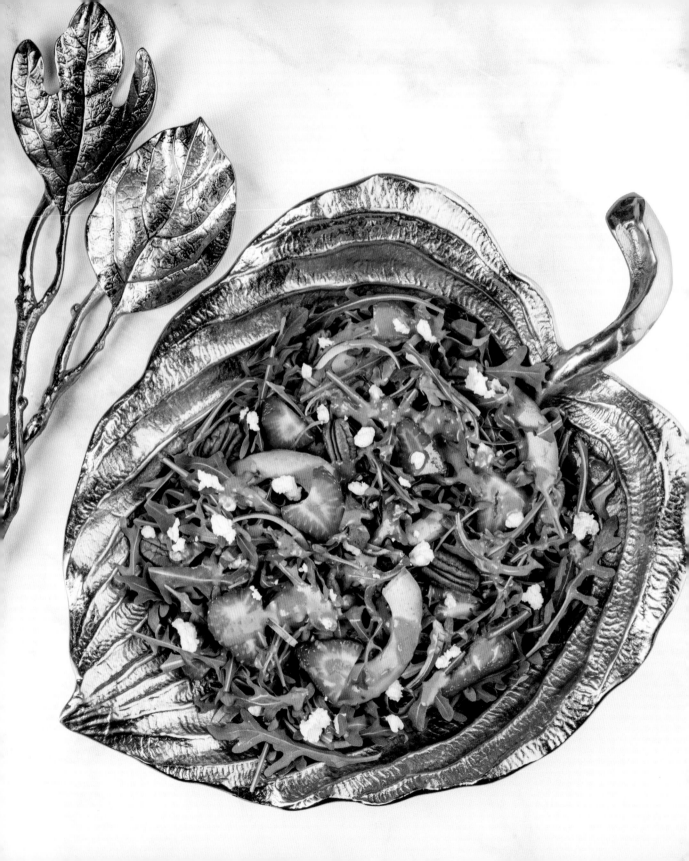

Arugula and Avocado Salad with Strawberry Dressing

This is an incredible summer salad packed with nutrients. The strawberries are a great source of antioxidants and fiber, which may have heart benefits and can help control blood sugar levels. The bright pink strawberry dressing is a bit tangy-sweet and instantly adds a beautiful aesthetic to the salad.

Makes 4 servings

2 cups (290 g) strawberries, divided

4 cups (80 g) arugula

¼ red onion, thinly sliced

1 avocado, thinly sliced

¼ cups (28 g) pecans

¼ cup (28 g) crumbled goat cheese

3 tbsp (45 ml) extra virgin olive oil

1 tbsp (15 ml) Dijon mustard

1 tbsp (15 ml) apple cider vinegar

Sea salt to taste

Slice 1 cup (145 g) of the strawberries. In a large bowl, toss the sliced strawberries with the arugula, red onion, avocado, roasted pecans and goat cheese.

Using a small food processor, pulse the remaining 1 cup (145 g) of strawberries, the olive oil, Dijon mustard, apple cider vinegar and sea salt. Blend until the mixture turns to a light purée. Drizzle the salad with half of the dressing and toss well to coat. Taste a bite of the salad to determine if it needs more dressing. Transfer to a platter and serve.

> Nedi's Tip: *If you have time, roast the pecans in the oven or toast them in a dry skillet. It adds a delicious layer of flavor and crunch to the salad.*
>
> *If there is leftover dressing, it can be stored in the fridge for a week and served with grilled chicken or eaten as a dip with veggies.*

Buckwheat Salad with Arugula and Feta

This buckwheat salad is packed with so many nutrients. It can be eaten on its own as a light meal or accompanied by grilled shrimp or chicken. Buckwheat is a superfood and is actually a seed that is similar to grain but completely free of gluten. It has a rich, nutty flavor and it's great for those who are intolerant to wheat. Due to its high fiber content, buckwheat improves digestion (prevents constipation) and may help to control blood sugar levels. Though not gluten free, farro, spelt or barley can be used if you don't have buckwheat.

Makes 4 servings

Salad

⅔ cups (112 g) dry buckwheat

2 cups (40 g) arugula

1 Persian cucumber, chopped

1 yellow bell pepper, chopped

1 cup (150 g) cherry tomatoes, sliced in half

½ cup (82 g) canned chickpeas, drained and rinsed

3 green onions, finely chopped

2 tbsp (8 g) finely chopped fresh mint

2 tbsp (8 g) finely chopped fresh parsley

¼ cup (38 g) crumbled feta cheese

Dressing

3 tbsp (45 ml) fresh lemon juice

2 tbsp (30 ml) extra virgin olive oil

1 clove garlic, minced

½ tsp dried oregano

½ tsp cumin

Sea salt and pepper to taste

Cook the buckwheat per the package instructions. When cooked, drain the buckwheat and place it in a large mixing bowl. Set aside to cool for 10 minutes.

Add the arugula, cucumber, bell pepper, cherry tomatoes, chickpeas, green onions, mint, parsley and feta to the cooled buckwheat.

In a small bowl, whisk the lemon juice, olive oil, garlic, oregano, cumin, salt and pepper until well combined. Pour the dressing over the salad and gently toss until all the flavors mix and everything is evenly combined.

> **Nedi's Tips:** *Try adding roasted red peppers instead of a bell pepper to switch up the flavors.*
>
> *This salad can be stored in the fridge for up to 3 days.*

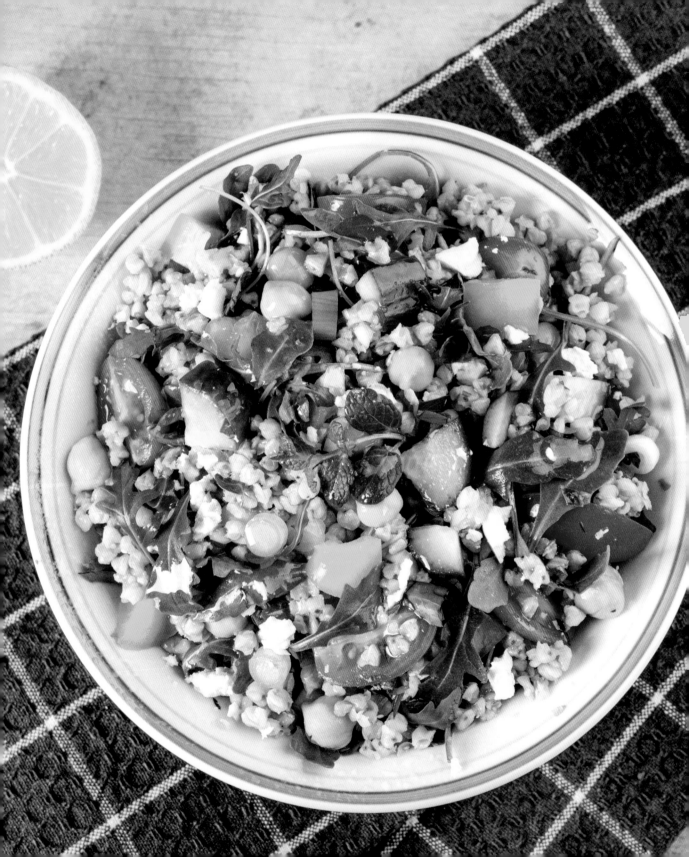

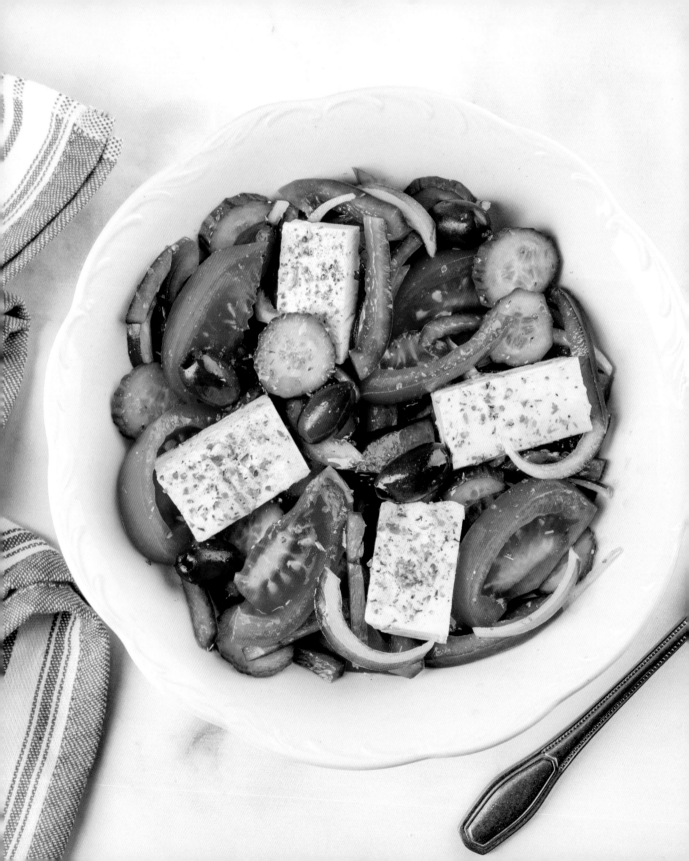

Traditional Greek Salad

If you love an authentic Greek salad, this recipe will make you feel like you are eating at a taverna on one of the gorgeous islands in Greece. Each bite of this refreshing salad will take your taste buds to the flavors of the Mediterranean. Greek salad is known as horiatiki, which means village salad. It means that it's a simple, rustic dish and the vegetables are thrown into a bowl, without needing a fancy preparation. This salad can be served with almost any dish or eaten on its own as a lighter midday meal.

Makes 4 servings

2 medium ripe tomatoes, cut into wedges

2 Persian cucumbers, sliced

½ red onion, thinly sliced

½ small green bell pepper, thinly sliced

3 tbsp (45 ml) extra virgin olive oil, divided

1 tbsp (15 ml) apple cider vinegar

Sea salt, to taste

1 (7-oz [200-g]) block feta cheese

6 Kalamata olives

½ tsp dried oregano

Place the tomatoes, cucumber, onion and bell pepper in a shallow bowl. Drizzle with 2 tablespoons (30 ml) of the olive oil and sprinkle with the apple cider vinegar. Season with salt to taste.

Cut the feta into four squares and spread in the bowl. Top the salad with the olives.

Drizzle the remaining 1 tablespoon (15 ml) of olive oil over the feta and sprinkle with the oregano.

> **Nedi's Tips:** *Find ripe, juicy tomatoes to make this salad even better!*
>
> *Red wine vinegar can be used in place of apple cider if you'd prefer or don't have apple cider vinegar on hand.*

Roasted Beet Salad with Goat Cheese

This is a great fall starter for a dinner party. The roasted beets get extra flavor from the creamy goat cheese and tangy orange–balsamic dressing. If you want to make a heartier meal out of this salad, try adding ½ cup (100 g) of cooked quinoa or farro or top it with grilled chicken.

Makes 4 servings

Salad
5 red beets

½ bunch (6–7 spears) asparagus, ends trimmed

4 cups (80 g) arugula

¼ cup (28 g) crumbled goat cheese

¼ cup (28 g) walnuts, finely chopped

Dressing
2 tbsp (30 ml) balsamic vinegar

½ orange, juiced

2 tbsp (30 ml) extra virgin olive oil

1 tsp honey or maple syrup

Sea salt and pepper to taste

Preheat the oven to 400°F (205°C). Tightly wrap each beet in foil and place on a baking sheet. Bake for 50 to 60 minutes, until the beets are tender. Poke a hole into a beet with a fork or knife to test them (when tender the fork/knife should easily slide in) before removing from the oven. Larger beets may need an extra 10 minutes or so. Let them cool until you can handle them, then peel them and cut them into wedges.

Meanwhile, bring a pot of water to a boil. Prepare a large bowl of water with ice and set it near the stove. Cook the asparagus in the boiling water for 3 minutes, until it is crisp-tender. Use tongs to transfer the asparagus directly to the ice bath to prevent it from overcooking. Once cooled, cut the asparagus spears into 2-inch (5-cm) pieces.

Place the arugula in a large serving bowl and add the beet wedges, asparagus pieces, goat cheese and walnuts.

In a small mixing bowl, combine the balsamic vinegar, orange juice, olive oil, honey, salt and pepper for the dressing. Mix well and lightly drizzle most of the dressing over the salad. Toss gently, taste and add more dressing if needed, then serve.

> **Nedi's Tips:** *If the beets have the greens on top, save them for soups or add them to a juicer along with other greens.*
>
> *If you are in a rush and want to save time, buy pre-roasted beets and simply toss them into the salad.*

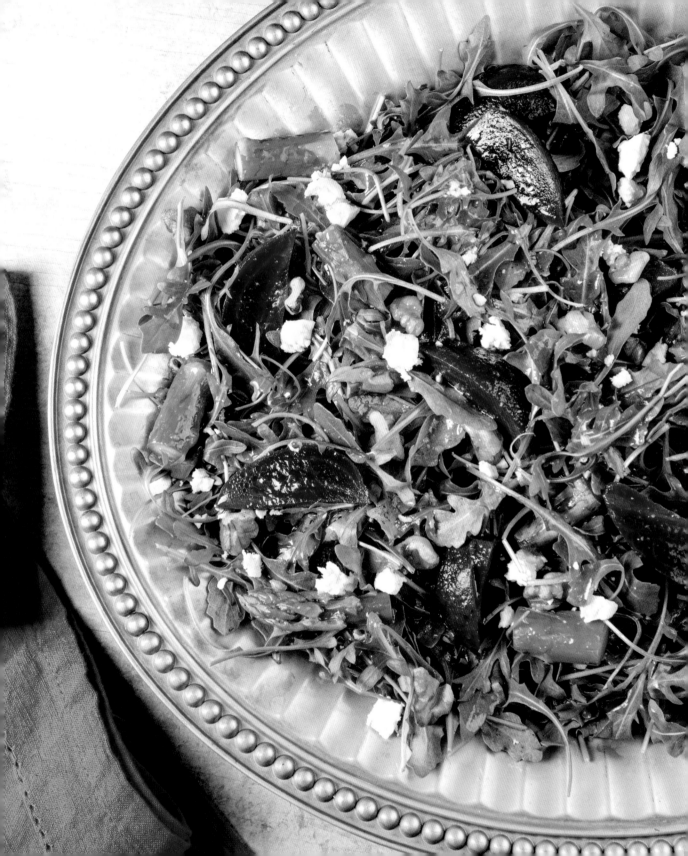

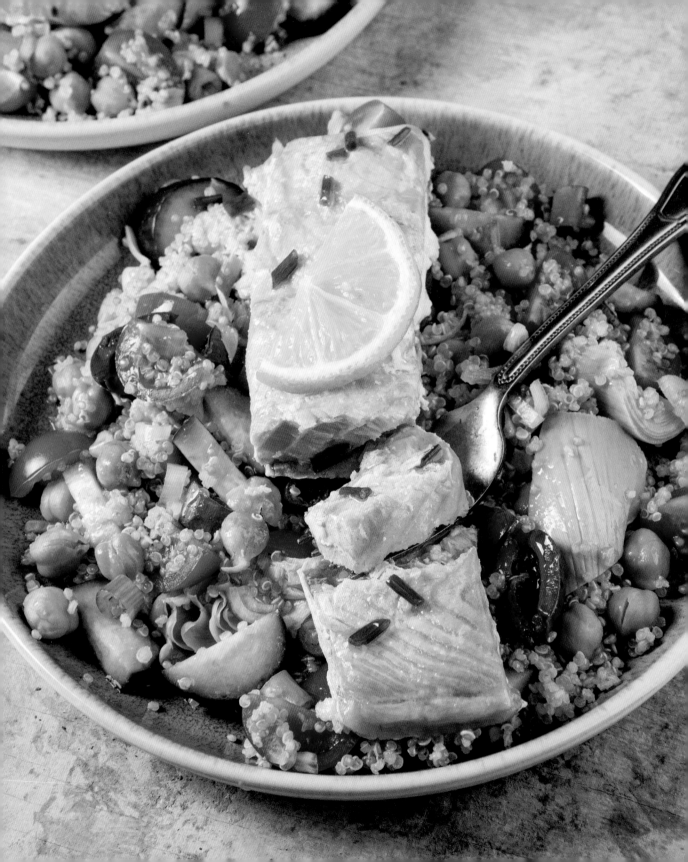

Delicacies from the Sea

Fresh seafood is one of the cornerstones of a Mediterranean diet. High in omega-3 fatty acids, protein and vitamin D, seafood is a main reason that this way of eating is so healthy. From Quick and Easy Shrimp Saganaki (page 71) to Oven Roasted Sea Bream (page 67) and Spaghetti alle Vongole (page 83), these dishes will make you feel like you're dining alongside the mesmerizing Mediterranean Sea. Choose fresh, high-quality fish to bring out the best natural flavors in your seafood dishes.

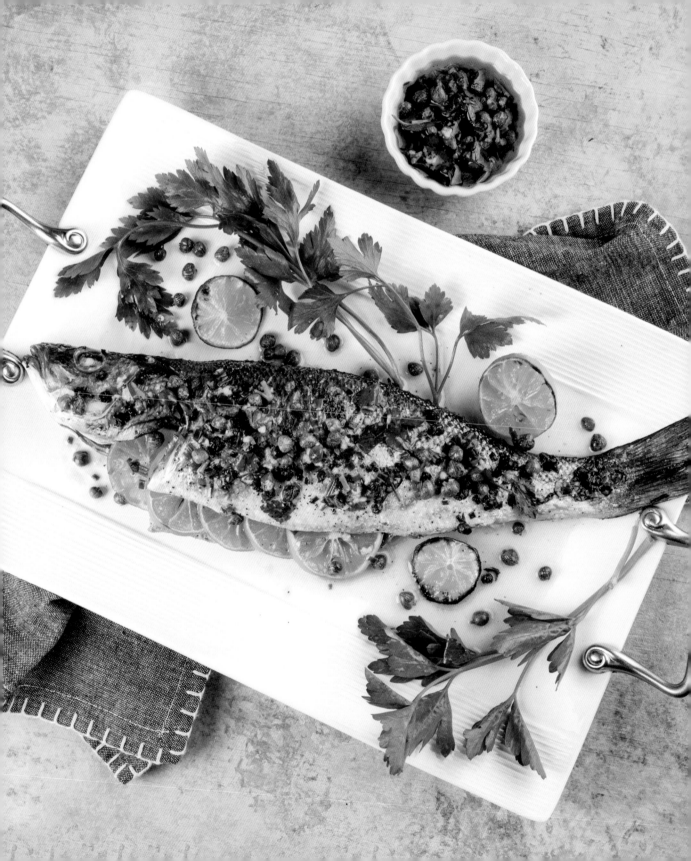

Oven Roasted Sea Bream

This is a classic family recipe that we always make in the summer months. Sea bream (tsipoura in Greek) is a flavorful fish that is rich in omega-3 fatty acids, vitamins and minerals, making it a great choice to include in your diet. Baking it in the oven really brings out the flavors and will make you feel like you are dining right on the Mediterranean. This oven roasted fish tastes divine when paired with Broccolini with Garlic, Lemon Zest and Feta (page 137).

Makes 4 servings

2 lb 2 oz (1 kg) whole sea bream, washed and cleaned (see Nedi's Tip)

Sea salt and pepper

⅓ cup (80 ml) extra virgin olive

¼ cup (60 ml) fresh lemon juice

¼ cup (15 g) parsley

2 tbsp (6 g) chopped chives

3 tbsp (25 g) capers

2 cloves garlic, minced

1 lemon

Preheat the oven to 400°F (205°C).

Line a baking dish with parchment paper and place the whole fish on top. Lightly salt and pepper the fish on each side and on the insides.

In a mixing bowl, whisk together the olive oil, lemon juice, parsley, chives, capers and garlic. Pour half of it over the fish, massaging the insides and both sides. (Save the other half of the mixture to pour over the fish once it is served.)

Cut the lemon in half. Slice half of it and place the slices inside of the fish. Cut the other half into wedges and reserve for garnish.

Add ½ cup (120 ml) of water to the baking dish. Cover the dish with foil and bake for 25 minutes. Remove the foil and continue baking for another 15 minutes. Take the fish out of the baking dish and set it aside to cool. Save any remaining sauce from the pan and place it in a small bowl.

When the fish has cooled, debone it and serve. Top the fish with the reserved lemon dressing and add a drizzle of the sauce it cooked in.

> Nedi's Tip: *This recipe works with many different types of white fish. I personally love it with Mediterranean sea bass, which is sold under various names including branzino and loup de mer.*

Greek-Style Salmon Kebabs with Dill and Garlic

I am a big fan of salmon. It is low in mercury and packed full of healthy omega-3 fatty acids, which are so great for healthy skin, hair and nails. Eating a diet rich in omega-3s helps to fight inflammation in the body.

This is a very healthy, light and refreshing recipe. The marinade keeps the salmon juicy, and the dill adds a delicious, earthy and slightly tangy taste. This Greek-style salmon with tzatziki will transport you to Greece while you are still at home.

Makes 4 servings

3 tbsp (45 ml) extra virgin olive oil, divided, plus more for greasing

Zest and juice from ½ lemon

1 tbsp (15 ml) plain Greek yogurt

1 clove garlic, grated

¼ cup (13 g) chopped fresh dill

14 oz (400 g) salmon, skinless and cut into bite-sized cubes

Sea salt and pepper

1 green bell pepper, cut into cubes

1 batch Refreshing Tzatziki (page 145), for serving

1 batch Baby Potatoes with Garlic and Dill (page 134), for serving

In a small bowl, combine 1 tablespoon (15 ml) of the olive oil, the lemon zest, lemon juice, yogurt, garlic and dill. Mix well. Season the salmon cubes with salt and pepper. Marinate the salmon with the sauce and refrigerate for 30 to 60 minutes.

To assemble the kebabs, thread a piece of marinated salmon on a metal skewer and follow it with a cube of green bell pepper. Repeat, alternating each salmon cube with a pepper cube until you have about three of each per skewer.

Coat a grill pan with a bit of olive oil to prevent sticking. Baste each kebab with the remaining 2 tablespoons (30 ml) of olive oil and grill over high heat for 2 to 3 minutes per side (about 8 minutes in total) until the salmon is cooked through.

Serve the salmon kebabs hot with the Refreshing Tzatziki and warm Baby Potatoes with Garlic and Dill.

> Nedi's Tip: *If you are not a fan of dill, try this recipe with parsley or cilantro.*

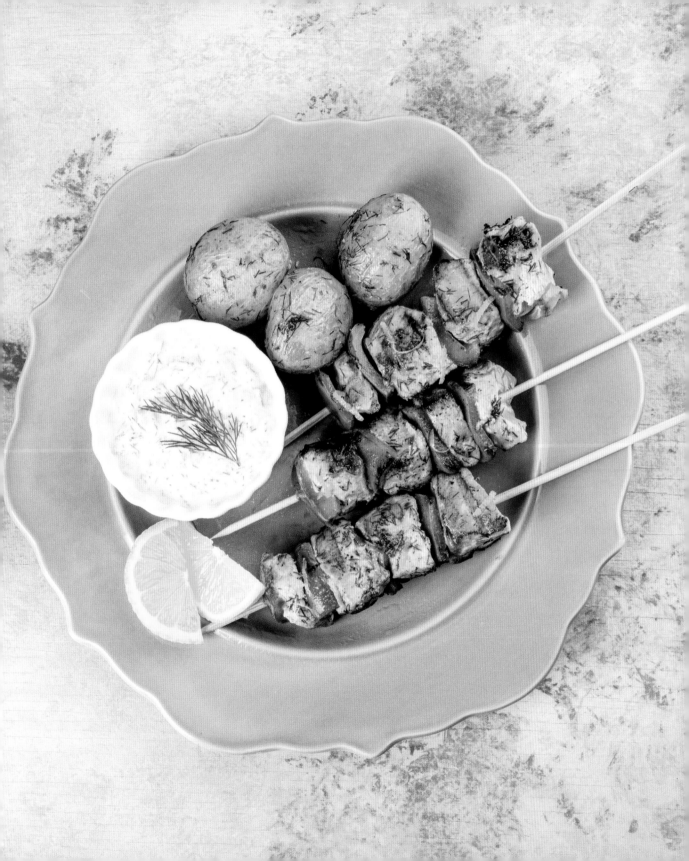

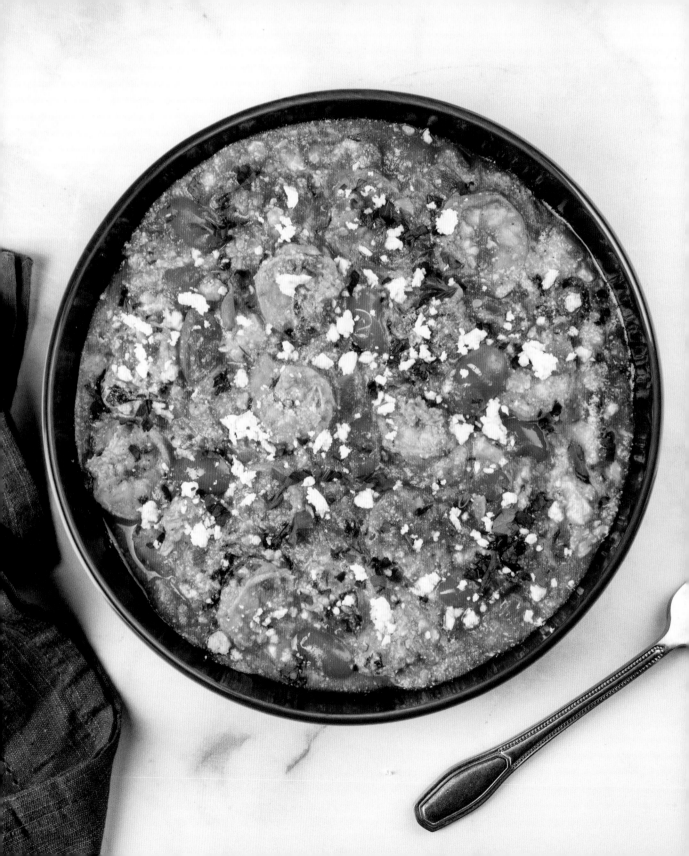

Quick and Easy Shrimp Saganaki

Shrimp saganaki is a classic Greek dish that the whole family will love. The most common saganaki recipes can be made with cheese, shrimp or mussels. The name of the dish comes from sagani, a type of frying pan that has two handles, making it easy to serve the dish. I love using a cast-iron pan for this recipe, but any frying pan will do just fine if it fits all the ingredients. This delicious, spicy, rich and creamy dish is super easy to make, and you can have dinner ready in under 30 minutes. Serve it with toasted pita bread, Traditional Greek Salad (page 61) and a chilled glass of ouzo or white wine. Cheers!

Makes 4 servings

¼ cup (60 ml) extra virgin olive oil

1 small red onion, finely diced

1 green pepper, chopped

1 cup (150 g) cherry or grape tomatoes, cut in half

3 cloves garlic, minced

¼ tsp chili flakes

1 tsp dried oregano

1½ cups (360 ml) crushed tomatoes

1 tsp sea salt

½ tsp pepper

1 lb (454 g) large shrimp, peeled and deveined

¼ cup (60 ml) white wine

1 cup (150 g) crumbled feta cheese

2 tbsp (12 g) chopped fresh mint, for garnish

2 tbsp (8 g) chopped fresh parsley, for garnish

Heat the olive oil in a large cast-iron pan or skillet over medium heat and cook the onion for 2 to 3 minutes, until translucent. Add the green pepper, cherry tomatoes, garlic, chili flakes and oregano and cook for 2 minutes.

Add the crushed tomatoes, salt and pepper. Cook for 5 minutes, until the sauce starts to thicken. Add the shrimp and white wine. Stir, cover the skillet and cook for 4 minutes on medium-low.

Uncover the skillet and sprinkle with the feta. Bring the heat to low and cover with a lid. Cook for 3 to 5 more minutes until the feta starts to soften.

Uncover the skillet and remove it from the heat. Garnish the shrimp saganaki with chopped mint and parsley and enjoy!

> Nedi's Tip: *If you are using frozen shrimp, either defrost them the night before in the refrigerator or place them in a bowl of cold water for an hour or two until fully defrosted.*

Mediterranean Halibut en Papillote

This is a light and elegant meal that is ideal during the warm months. This recipe seems fancier than it is. The fish is simply poached in a parchment pouch with fresh vegetables and herbs for flavor. The dish should be served in the pouches as it will release a divine aroma when you open up the pouch. Pair with a side of Greek Spinach Rice (page 133) and a glass of crisp white wine and enjoy!

Makes 2 servings

2 (6-oz [170-g]) filets of halibut

Sea salt and pepper to taste

10 cherry tomatoes, sliced in half

½ shallot, thinly sliced

½ cup (90 g) Kalamata olives, pitted and sliced in half

2 tbsp (17 g) capers

2 tbsp (8 g) chopped parsley

¼ cup (60 ml) white wine

¼ cup (60 ml) extra virgin olive oil

½ lemon, thinly sliced

Preheat the oven to 400°F (205°C). Pat the fish dry and sprinkle with salt and pepper. Set aside.

Fold a piece of parchment paper in half. Place the fish filet on one side of the parchment paper and cover with half of the cherry tomatoes, shallot, olives, capers, parsley, white wine and olive oil. Place half of the lemon slices on top and reserve the rest for garnish.

Fold the other half of the parchment paper over and seal the edges making a small fold every ½ inch (1.3 cm) all the way around to create a half-moon shape. Repeat with the other piece of parchment and remaining ingredients.

Place both pouches on a baking sheet. Bake for 15 to 20 minutes, until the parchment paper has puffed up and the fish is flaky and cooked through.

> Nedi's Tip: *This recipe works well with a variety of fileted fish like halibut, cod, branzino or sole.*

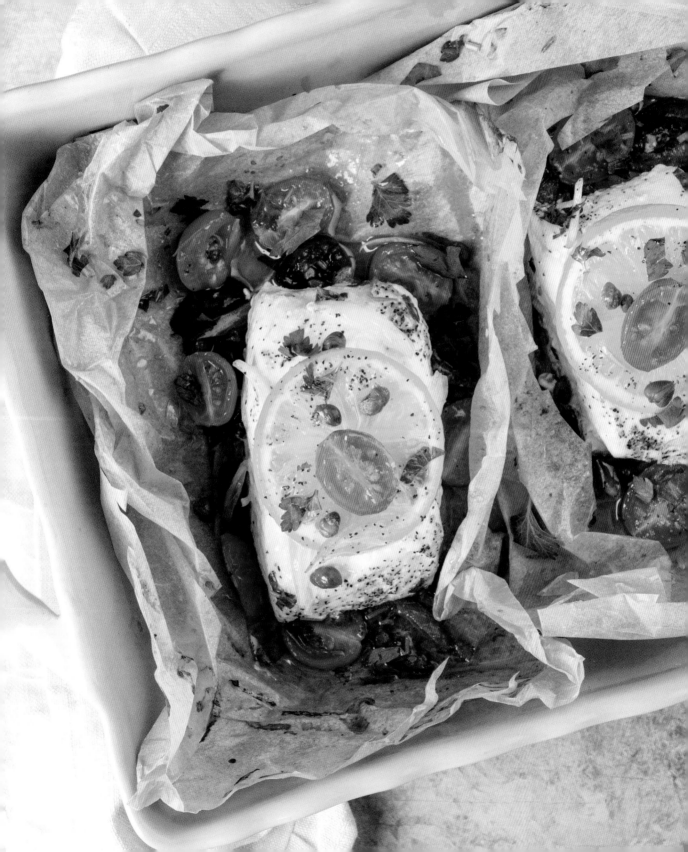

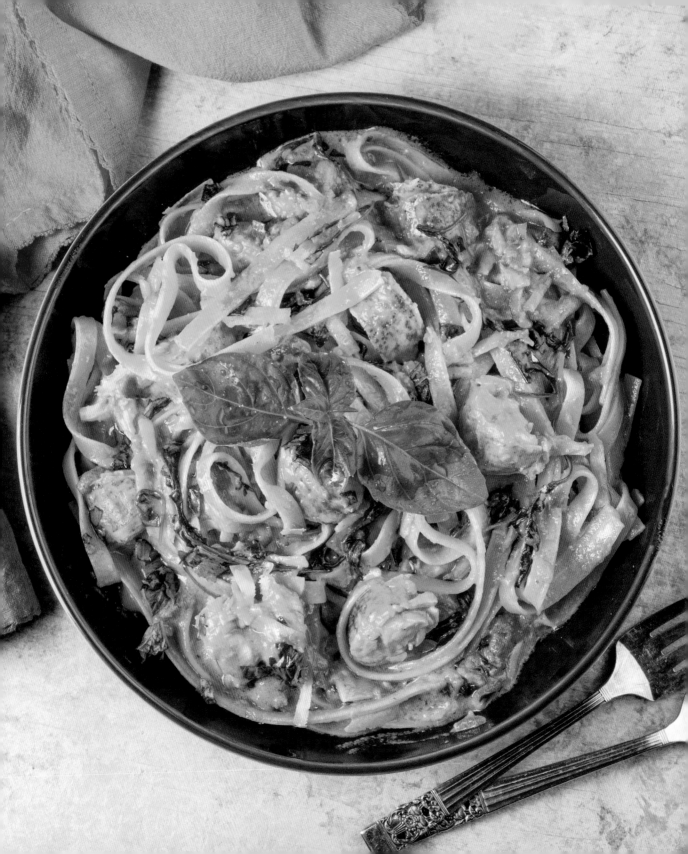

Fettuccine with Pink Lobster Sauce

This lobster fettuccine is always a hit in our household. It's a beautiful pasta dish that is easier to make than it sounds. The lobster only cooks for 5 minutes but many stores sell precooked lobster if you prefer that. Whenever I am in a Greek restaurant and I see lobster pasta on the menu, I get so excited and always order it. Try this dish and let the flavors take you to the Mediterranean.

Makes 4 servings

1 tsp sea salt

4 lobster tails or 2 cups (340 g) cooked lobster meat

8 oz (226 g) dried fettuccine pasta

2 tbsp (30 ml) extra virgin olive oil

2 shallots, chopped

3 cloves garlic, minced

½ tsp chili flakes

½ cup (120 ml) coconut cream

2 cups (480 ml) tomato sauce

Sea salt and pepper to taste

2 cups (40 g) arugula

6 tbsp (38 g) grated pecorino Romano

3 tbsp (8 g) chopped fresh basil

Fill a pot of water with the salt and bring to a boil. Cook the lobster tails for 5 minutes. Remove the lobster from the water and rinse with cold water. Separate the meat from the tail and chop it into ½-inch (1.3-cm) chunks.

Meanwhile, bring a separate pot of water to a boil and cook the fettuccine per the package instructions.

Heat the olive oil in a large skillet over medium heat and sauté the shallots for 2 minutes. Add the garlic and chili flakes and cook for another minute.

Add the coconut cream and tomato sauce and season with salt and pepper to taste. Add the lobster meat and arugula and stir to coat. Cook for 1 minute to warm the lobster and wilt the arugula, then turn off the heat.

Drain the fettuccine, reserving ½ cup (120 ml) of the pasta water, and transfer the pasta to the skillet with the sauce. Sprinkle the pecorino Romano over the pasta and stir to coat the pasta. Add some of the reserved pasta water if the sauce is too thick. Stir in the basil, toss once more, and serve immediately.

> *Nedi's Tip: The lobster tail requires the use of strong kitchen scissors to cut through, so if you don't have those I recommend purchasing cooked lobster if it's available in the grocery store.*

Seared Scallops with Pesto and Zucchini Noodles

This dairy-free, vegan pesto is just as good as traditional pesto. The combination of basil and pine nuts adds tons of flavor while minimizing calories—I promise you won't miss the Parmesan cheese once you try this! The sauce pairs so well with the garlicky pan-seared scallops. This recipe is very flexible. The pesto can be made with any nuts of your choice and the basil can be swapped for kale, spinach or arugula.

Zucchini noodles are a great substitute for carb-heavy pasta. If you are watching your weight, this is a great swap. One cup of zucchini noodles has about 40 calories compared to regular spaghetti, which has about 200 calories per cup. Zoodles also provide a good amount of nutrients like vitamin C, vitamin A, several B vitamins and potassium.

Makes 2 servings

Vegan Pesto

2 cups (48 g) tightly packed whole basil leaves

2 cloves garlic

½ cup (60 g) pine nuts

¼ cup (60 ml) extra virgin olive oil

3 tbsp (45 ml) fresh lime juice

Sea salt to taste

Zucchini Noodles and Scallops

3 zucchini, ends trimmed

4 tbsp (60 ml) extra virgin olive oil, divided

2 tbsp (28 g) butter, divided

8–10 large scallops (about 8 oz [226 g]), washed and patted dry

Sea salt and pepper to taste

2 cloves garlic, minced

1 tbsp (3 g) finely chopped fresh dill

¼ tsp chili flakes

2 tbsp (30 ml) fresh lemon juice

To make the pesto, in a food processor, combine the basil leaves, garlic, pine nuts, olive oil, lime juice and salt. Pulse until well combined.

To make the noodles, spiralize into zucchini noodles using a vegetable spiralizer. Trim the noodles with scissors so they aren't too long.

Heat 1 tablespoon (15 ml) of olive oil in a large skillet over medium heat. Add the zucchini noodles and sauté for 2 minutes. Toss in the pesto sauce and mix it well into the noodles using tongs. Cook for 2 minutes and set aside.

For the scallops, in a smaller skillet, heat 2 tablespoons (30 ml) of the olive oil and 1 tablespoon (14 g) of butter. Add the scallops and season with sea salt and pepper to your taste. Cook for a minute on each side and remove from the skillet.

Add the remaining 1 tablespoon (15 ml) olive oil and butter to the skillet. Add the garlic and cook for 1 minute. Turn off the heat and add the scallops, dill, chili flakes and lemon juice. Toss well, making sure the scallops are covered on each side. Divide the zucchini noodles between two plates and top with scallops. Enjoy!

Nedi's Tip: *I love the flavor that lime juice lends to the pesto, but if needed it can be substituted for lemon juice.*

If you are not a big fan of zucchini noodles, try using gluten-free spaghetti or spaghetti squash.

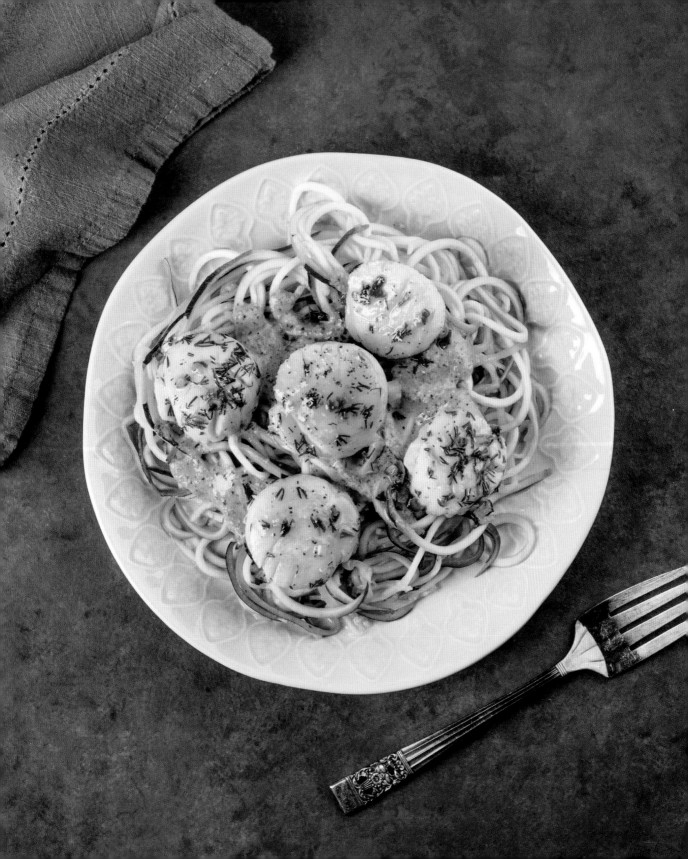

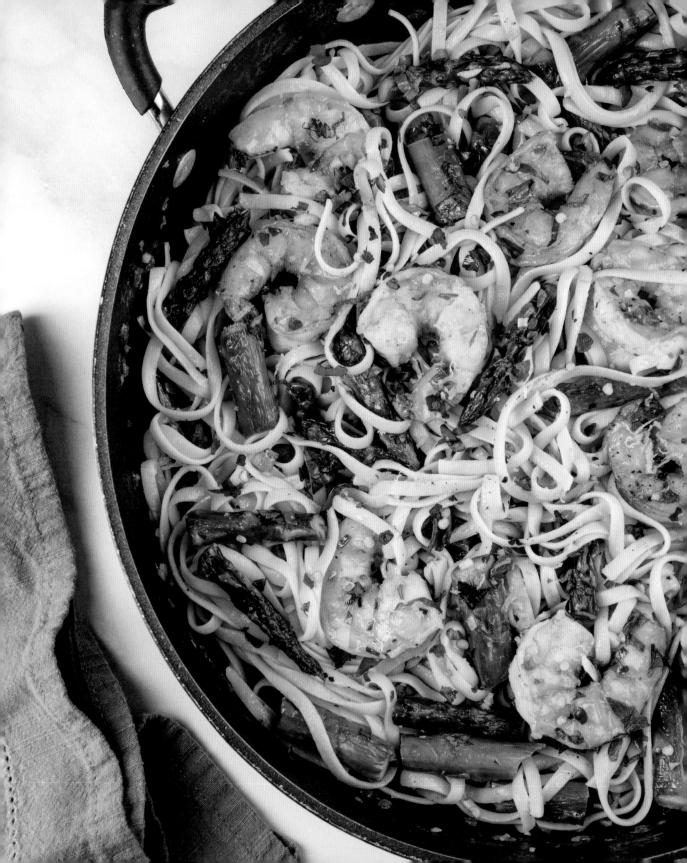

Shrimp Scampi Linguine

This classic pasta dish is the ultimate crowd-pleaser. It's light, buttery and so delicious. I love the addition of asparagus. The asparagus pairs so well with the shrimp and boosts the nutrients of the dish. Asparagus is a great source of fiber, folate, potassium and vitamins A, C and K.

This recipe doesn't require much time to prepare and makes a beautiful dinner. I typically make it with linguine, but spaghetti or angel hair can be used as well. The pasta used is entirely up to you; a gluten-free pasta will taste good and so would a pasta substitute such as zucchini noodles.

Makes 6 servings

10.5 oz (300 g) linguine

3 tbsp (45 ml) extra virgin olive oil, divided

3 tbsp (42 g) butter, divided

½ lb (226 g) asparagus, trimmed and cut into 2-inch (5-cm) pieces

1 red onion, finely chopped

4 cloves garlic, minced

¼ tsp chili flakes

Sea salt and pepper to taste

1 lb (454 g) raw shrimp, peeled and deveined

1 cup (240 ml) dry white wine

Juice and zest of 1 lemon

½ cup (32 g) finely chopped fresh parsley

In a large pot, cook the linguine according to package instructions. Save ½ cup (120 ml) of the pasta water and drain the linguine.

Heat 1 tablespoon (15 ml) of the olive oil and 1 tablespoon (14 g) of the butter in a large skillet over medium-high heat. Add the asparagus and cook for 5 minutes, stirring occasionally. Remove the asparagus from the skillet and set aside.

Using the same hot skillet, heat the remaining 2 tablespoons (30 ml) of olive oil and 2 tablespoons (28 g) of butter. Add the onion and cook for 2 minutes, until translucent. Add the garlic and chili flakes to the skillet and cook for another minute.

Season the shrimp with salt and pepper and add to the skillet. Cook for 2 to 3 minutes, until the shrimp are pink and no longer translucent. Remove the shrimp from the skillet and set aside so they don't overcook.

Add the white wine, a little bit of the pasta water and the lemon juice to the skillet. Bring to a boil and turn off the heat. Toss in the cooked linguine, asparagus, shrimp and parsley. Mix gently until well coated. Garnish with the lemon zest and serve.

> Nedi's Tips: *Try this recipe using red lentil spaghetti to boost the nutritional value.*
>
> *The asparagus can be swapped out with broccolini.*

Veggie-Packed Quinoa Salad with Roasted Salmon

This is a beautiful salad, packed with vitamins, antioxidants, fiber and protein. The quinoa salad can be made ahead of time and stays fresh in the fridge for 2 to 3 days. It is perfect for meal prep since you can portion it in individual serving containers either for quick dinners during the week or to bring to work for lunch. I also like to add feta cheese and skip the salmon if I am in a rush. Plus, if you pre-cook the quinoa the day before, the dish comes together very easily within 15 minutes.

Makes 4 servings

Quinoa Salad

½ cup (90 g) uncooked quinoa

1 English cucumber, seeded and cut into quarter-moons

1 cup (150 g) cherry tomatoes, cut in half

1 cup (165 g) canned chickpeas, rinsed and drained

1 cup (240 g) marinated jarred artichoke hearts, cut in quarters

⅓ cup (40 g) Kalamata olives, pitted

½ shallot, thinly sliced

2 green onions, thinly sliced

¼ cup (25 g) finely chopped fresh mint

2 tbsp (30 ml) extra virgin olive oil

¼ cup (60 ml) fresh lemon juice

1 tsp sumac

Sea salt to taste

Roasted Salmon

4 (4-oz [113-g]) salmon filets

2 tbsp (30 ml) fresh lemon juice

2 tbsp (6 g) lemon zest

¼ cup (60 ml) extra virgin olive oil

2 tbsp (6 g) chopped chives

2 tsp (2 g) dried thyme

2 cloves garlic, minced

Sea salt and pepper to taste

To make the salad, cook the quinoa per package instructions. When cooked, set aside to cool for 10 minutes.

In a large bowl, combine the cucumber, cherry tomatoes, chickpeas, artichoke hearts, olives, shallots, green onions and the mint. Add the cooled quinoa and toss to combine all the ingredients.

In a small bowl, combine the olive oil, lemon juice, sumac and salt. Whisk to combine. Pour the dressing over the salad and mix well.

Meanwhile, preheat the oven to 425°F (220°C). Line a baking sheet with parchment paper and place the salmon on the parchment-lined sheet.

In a small bowl, combine the lemon juice, lemon zest, olive oil, chives, thyme, garlic, salt and pepper. Mix well and spread evenly over each salmon filet. Bake the salmon for 10 minutes for medium-rare or 12 minutes for medium.

To assemble, divide the quinoa salad among four shallow bowls and place a salmon filet on top of each bowl.

Nedi's Tips: To make this salad vegan, skip the salmon and top it with tofu, tempeh or warm mushrooms.

The quinoa can be made ahead of time and stored in the fridge until ready to make the salad.

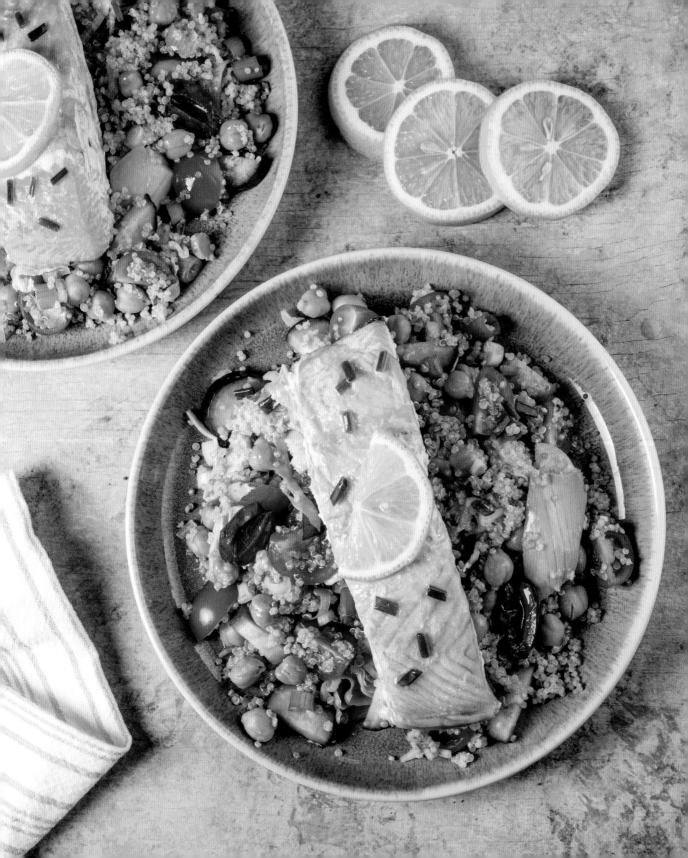

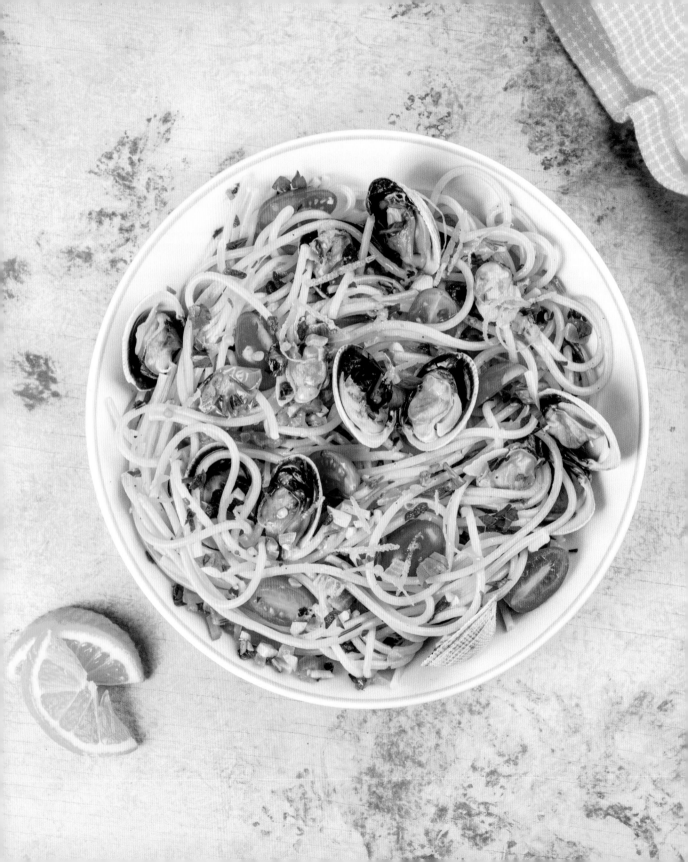

Spaghetti alle Vongole

Out of all the wonderful pasta dishes, spaghetti alle vongole is on top of my list for the best Italian pasta. The sauce is light and perfect for a hot summer night. Traditionally, the recipe is made with spaghetti, linguine or even fettuccine; keep in mind that Italians don't use short pasta for this dish. I am quite generous with the garlic and chili flakes, but feel free to use a little less if you don't like spicy heat. This pasta sauce can be made with or without tomatoes; I personally love the addition of fresh cherry tomatoes!

Makes 4 servings

½ lb (226 g) spaghetti

2 lb (907 g) clams, such as cockles or littleneck, rinsed and drained

4 tbsp (60 ml) extra virgin olive oil, divided

1 shallot, finely chopped

5 cloves garlic, finely chopped

1 tsp chili flakes

1 cup (150 g) cherry tomatoes, sliced in half

Sea salt and pepper to taste

½ cup (120 ml) dry white wine

1 cup (60 g) fresh parsley, finely chopped

Zest and juice of ½ lemon

Boil the spaghetti per package instructions. Reserve ½ cup (120 ml) of the pasta water and drain the rest.

In a large pot over medium heat, cook the clams for about 2 minutes, covered, until they start to open. Discard any that didn't open. Transfer them to a bowl and save the juice that they released. Using a fine strainer, strain the clam juice to remove sand residue. Remove half of the clams from their shells using a fork and discard the shells. This step isn't required but I find it easier to eat and the shells won't overpower the serving plate.

Heat 2 tablespoons (30 ml) of the olive oil in a large skillet over medium heat. Add the shallot, garlic and chili flakes. Cook until the shallot and garlic are golden, then add the cherry tomatoes and season with salt and pepper to your taste. Pour in the white wine and add the clams and clam juice to the pan. Cover and cook for 2 to 3 minutes.

Add the drained spaghetti to the skillet and toss with the sauce and clams. Add the reserved pasta cooking water and stir in the chopped parsley (reserve a small amount for garnishing), lemon zest and lemon juice. Drizzle with the remaining 2 tablespoons (30 ml) of the olive oil, toss once more and plate. Garnish with remaining parsley and enjoy!

> Nedi's Tip: *For a low-carb version, try this recipe with hearts of palm spaghetti or spaghetti squash.*

Sea Bass Lettuce Wraps

Nothing tastes better than a light and fresh seafood meal in the summertime. The fish in this recipe can be grilled, pan-grilled or baked in the oven. These fish "tacos" are served in lettuce cups with crunchy cabbage and are absolutely divine. They are light, refreshing and flavorful.

Makes 4 servings

Sea Bass

2 (1.3-lb [600-g]) filets sea bass, skinless

1 small orange, juiced (about ⅓ cup [80 ml])

1 tbsp (15 ml) extra virgin olive oil

½ lime, juiced

Sea salt and pepper to taste

Cabbage Topping

2 cups (140 g) purple cabbage, thinly sliced

1 small red onion, thinly sliced

1 jalapeño, thinly sliced

¼ cup (6 g) chopped cilantro

½ tsp sea salt

1 lime, juiced

1 tbsp (15 ml) extra virgin olive oil

Sauce

2 tbsp (30 ml) mayonnaise

2 tsp (10 ml) chili-garlic sauce, or more to taste

1 tbsp (15 ml) lime juice

For Serving

1 head Boston bib lettuce or iceberg lettuce

2 limes, cut into wedges

To make the sea bass, preheat the oven to 400°F (205°C). Line a baking dish with parchment paper and place the sea bass filets on the parchment-lined sheet.

In a small bowl, mix the orange juice, olive oil, lime, salt and pepper. Pour the mixture over the fish and place the pan in the oven. Bake the fish filets for 12 to 14 minutes, until flaky.

While the fish cooks, prepare the cabbage topping. In a medium bowl, mix the cabbage, red onion, jalapeño, cilantro, salt, lime juice and olive oil. Toss to combine.

Finally, make the sauce. In a bowl, whisk together the mayo, chili garlic sauce and lime juice. Taste and add more chili–garlic sauce to make the sauce spicier if desired.

To assemble the "tacos," fill a lettuce leaf with pieces of the fish, top with the cabbage topping and drizzle with the sauce. Serve with lime wedges.

> Nedi's Tip: *If you can't find sea bass, you can use any white fish, such as cod, halibut or mahi mahi.*

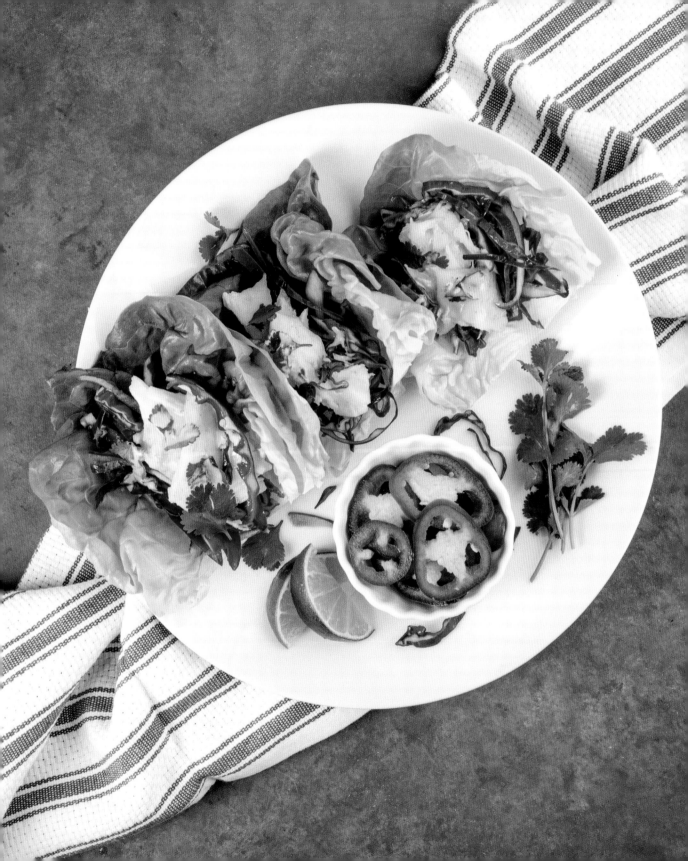

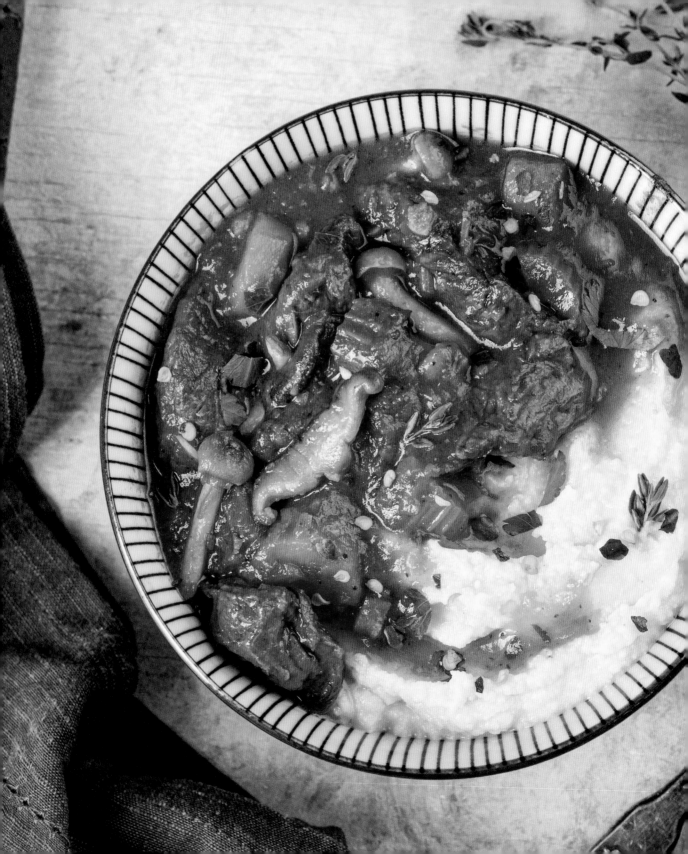

Comforting Dishes from the Land

One of the foundations of the Mediterranean diet is family-style meals made from lean meats sourced straight from the local farm. While I love these convivial meals, I find that they are oftentimes a little heavy for me. Over the past decade I've refined some of my favorite Mediterranean meat dishes with lower calorie and lower carb options. From Gluten-Free Crispy Chicken with Bruschetta-Style Salad (page 90) to Chicken Parm over Zucchini Noodles (page 93) to Low-Carb Lasagna with Mushrooms and Meat Ragu (page 97), these comforting meat dishes will satisfy and energize without leaving you feeling bloated or lethargic.

When purchasing protein, I like to think of how my grandmother shops—from a farmer or local butcher at the market. If I can, I purchase meat directly from a butcher. If that's not possible, I am conscious about the quality of the protein I buy from the grocery store, seeking out meat that carries third-party certifications such as certified humane and organic.

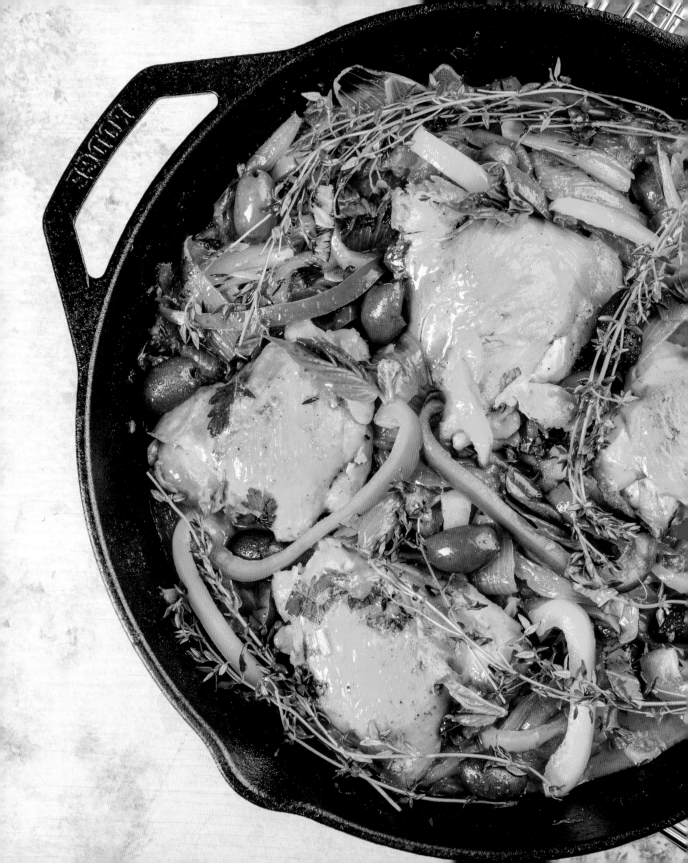

Juicy Mediterranean Chicken with Olives and Peppers

This is an impressive and light weeknight dinner that will be ready in under 30 minutes. It's perfect to make during the summer with beautiful, delicious, ripe tomatoes. In the winter, when tomatoes are not in season, I usually use canned diced tomatoes as store-bought fresh tomatoes won't be as tasty or nutrient-dense as in the summer months. This dish is full of flavor with a combination of classic Mediterranean ingredients—peppers, tomatoes, Kalamata olives, thyme and basil. Bell peppers add a lot of flavor and are an excellent source of vitamins A and C. Serve this dish with Low-Carb Potato–Cauliflower Mash (page 141).

Makes 6 servings

6 skinless and boneless chicken thighs

Sea salt and pepper

4 tbsp (60 ml) extra virgin olive oil, divided

5 medium shallots, peeled and quartered

1 green bell pepper, seeds removed and thinly sliced

1 yellow bell pepper, seeds removed and thinly sliced

1 red bell pepper, seeds removed and thinly sliced

¼ cup (60 ml) warm water or broth

5 cloves garlic, sliced

2 large tomatoes, diced (about 2 cups [360 g])

⅓ cup (80 ml) dry white wine

¼ tsp turmeric

12 sprigs fresh thyme

½ cup (60 g) pitted Kalamata olives

2 tbsp (6 g) chopped fresh basil, for garnish

2 tbsp (8 g) chopped fresh parsley, for garnish

Season the chicken with salt and pepper. Heat 2 tablespoons (30 ml) of the olive oil in a large skillet over medium heat then add the chicken. Cook for 3 to 4 minutes on each side, until the chicken is golden brown. Remove the chicken from the skillet and set aside.

Heat the remaining 2 tablespoons (30 ml) of the olive oil in the same skillet and then add the shallots and bell peppers. Cook for 2 to 3 minutes, stirring occasionally. Add the warm water or broth to prevent the shallots and peppers from sticking to the pan. Add the garlic and sauté for 1 minute. Add the tomatoes, white wine, turmeric and thyme. Bring to a boil. Reduce the heat to medium and simmer, covered, for 5 minutes.

Return the chicken thighs to the skillet and reduce the heat to low. Simmer, covered, stirring occasionally, for 25 minutes or until the chicken is cooked through (165°F [75°C] when checked with a meat thermometer). Add the Kalamata olives and simmer for another 5 minutes. Turn off heat and discard any large thyme sprigs from the sauce. Garnish with the fresh basil and parsley. Serve while hot.

Nedi's Tip: Chicken breast can be used if preferred.

Gluten-Free Crispy Chicken with Bruschetta-Style Salad

This gluten-free chicken is crispy on the outside and tender on the inside with no frying required. It tastes like it's been cooking for a long time and the seasonings have marinated beautifully. In reality, this meal can easily be thrown together at the last minute and it is perfection!

Makes 6 servings

3 large chicken breasts

1½ cups (145 g) almond meal/flour

Sea salt and pepper

1 tbsp (5 g) dried oregano

1 tsp cayenne pepper

1 tsp turmeric

2 eggs

2 cups (300 g) cherry tomatoes, sliced in half

1 clove garlic, minced

½ red onion, finely chopped

¼ cup (10 g) thinly sliced fresh basil leaves

2 tbsp (30 ml) balsamic vinegar

2 tbsp (30 ml) extra virgin olive oil

Sea salt to taste

4 cups (80 g) arugula

½ lemon

Slice each chicken breast in half horizontally so you have six thin pieces. Spread the almond meal/flour on a large plate and add the salt, pepper, oregano, cayenne and turmeric. Mix all the spices evenly into the almond meal/flour.

In a shallow bowl, crack the eggs and whisk. Dip each chicken breast into the egg mixture on each side and then into the almond crumb mix until all sides are well coated.

Meanwhile, preheat the oven to 425°F (220°C). Line a baking sheet with parchment paper and place each chicken breast on the parchment-lined baking sheet. Bake for 18 to 20 minutes, until cooked through and golden (165°F [75°C]).

To prepare the salad, add the cherry tomatoes, garlic, onion and basil to a bowl. Drizzle with the balsamic vinegar and olive oil and season to taste with salt. Toss until well combined.

Divide the arugula evenly among the six plates. Squeeze fresh lemon over the arugula then top with the chicken breast and bruschetta-style salad.

Nedi's Tip: This recipe can be made with veal instead of chicken and will taste just like veal Milanese—but is much healthier!

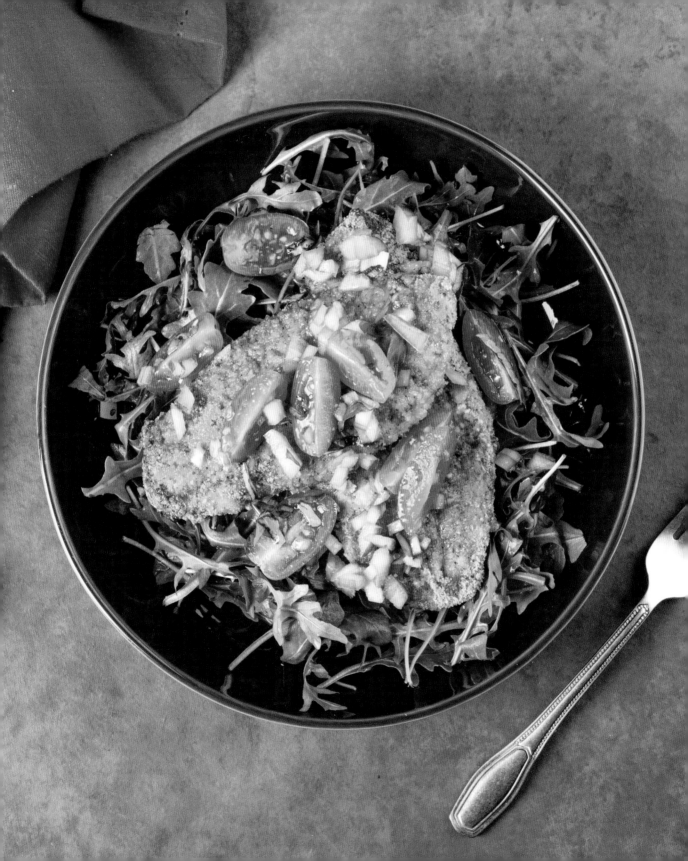

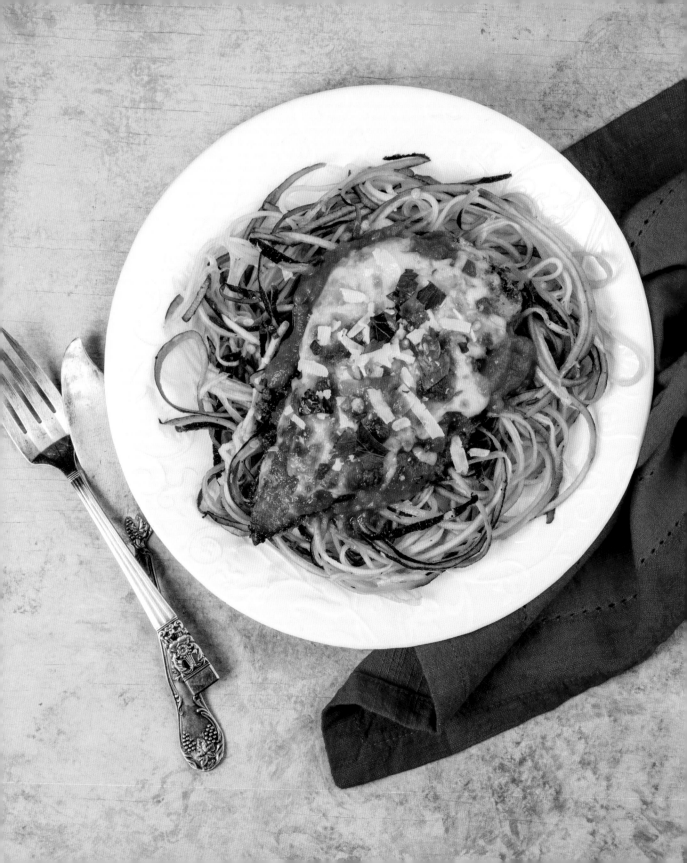

Chicken Parm over Zucchini Noodles

This is the best healthy version of the classic chicken parm you will ever taste! I have been making this recipe for years and some of my friends joke that it tastes better than the chicken parm at the well-known Italian restaurant Carbone. My version is gluten free and lightly breaded with a mix of almond meal/flour, aromatic spices and herbs. You can have this comforting meal ready in less than 30 minutes and satisfy those comfort-food cravings.

Makes 4 servings

1 egg

1 cup (95 g) almond meal/flour

1 tsp garlic powder

1 tsp paprika

1 tbsp (5 g) dried oregano

2 tbsp (8 g) chopped parsley

1 tbsp (18 g) sea salt

1 tsp pepper

2 chicken breasts, sliced in half horizontally to make four thin pieces

1 tbsp (15 ml) extra virgin olive oil

1½ cups (360 ml) tomato sauce, divided

1½ cup (168 g) shredded mozzarella

4 zucchini, spiralized

2 tbsp (15 g) pecorino Romano, grated

4 tsp (5 g) chopped fresh parsley, for garnish

Chili flakes, for garnish

Whisk the egg in a medium bowl and set aside. In a larger bowl, combine the almond meal/flour, garlic powder, paprika, oregano, parsley, sea salt and pepper.

Dip the four pieces of chicken breast into the egg wash and then dip each side into the almond mix.

Meanwhile, preheat the oven to 425°F (220°C) and line a baking sheet with parchment paper.

Heat the olive oil in a large skillet over medium heat then add the chicken. Sauté each side for 4 minutes, until golden. Place the chicken breasts evenly on the parchment-lined baking sheet and spread 1 to 2 tablespoons (15 to 30 ml) of tomato sauce over each breast. Top each chicken breast with some shredded mozzarella and bake for 15 minutes, until the cheese is melted and the chicken is cooked through (an internal temperature of 165°F [75°C]).

Spray a large skillet with cooking spray and sauté the zucchini noodles over medium heat. Add the remaining tomato sauce to the pan and toss with the grated pecorino Romano for extra flavor. Plate the zucchini noodles and top with the chicken breast. Garnish with parsley and chili flakes.

Nedi's Tip: Try baking the zucchini noodles in a baking dish mixed with tomato sauce and pecorino Romano. If you choose to bake the noodles, put them in the oven at the same time as the chicken so they cook for the same amount of time.

Pork Tenderloin in Creamy Mushroom Sauce

This tasty yet simple dish is a beautiful choice to serve when entertaining. The mushrooms, cooked in white wine and coconut cream with fresh thyme, add so much flavor to the tender pork. Serve it with Low-Carb Potato–Cauliflower Mash (page 141) or Baby Potatoes with Garlic and Dill (page 134).

Makes 4 servings

1 tbsp (15 ml) avocado oil

1 lb (454 g) pork tenderloin, cut into ½-inch (1.3-cm) pieces

Sea salt and pepper

1 tbsp (14 g) butter

1 lb (454 g) baby portobello mushrooms, sliced

2 cloves garlic, minced

½ cup (120 ml) dry white wine

3 sprigs fresh thyme, plus more for garnish

1 cup (240 ml) coconut cream

Heat the avocado oil in a skillet over medium to high heat and sprinkle the pork pieces with salt and pepper. Sear the pork tenderloin pieces on both sides, flipping them over several times, about 5 minutes total until they are well browned. It won't be cooked all the way yet because it will continue to cook after cooking the mushrooms. Transfer to a plate.

In the same skillet, heat the butter over medium heat and cook the mushrooms for 2 to 3 minutes. Add the garlic, stir to mix with the mushrooms then add the white wine and thyme. Cook for 2 minutes then stir in the coconut cream. Season with salt and pepper again to taste.

Add the meat back into the skillet and lower the heat. Cook, covered, for 10 minutes, until the sauce reduces. Insert a food thermometer into a piece of pork, it should read 145°F (63°C). Garnish with fresh thyme and serve.

Nedi's Tips: This recipe can easily be made with chicken breasts or thighs or beef steaks. The mushroom sauce pairs well with different meat and it is truly delicious.

You can also use any mushrooms you have on hand. This recipe will taste good with shiitake, cremini or white mushrooms.

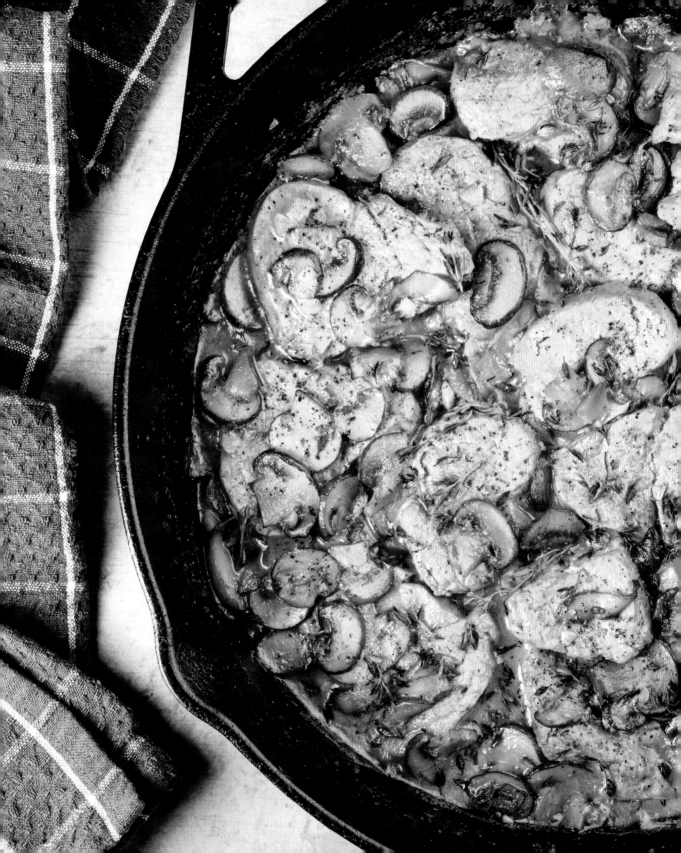

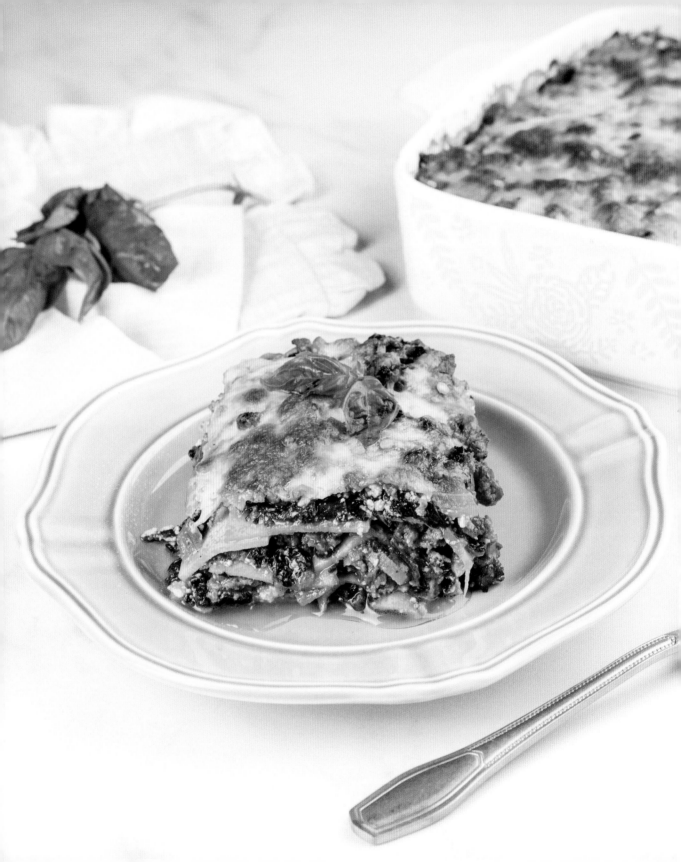

Low-Carb Lasagna with Mushrooms and Meat Ragu

This low carb lasagna tastes just like the real thing. It is so rich, and the combination of spices really elevates the flavors. I love using hearts of palm lasagna sheets for this recipe. If you aren't a fan of them or aren't able to get them, try it with lentil lasagna sheets or gluten-free lasagna sheets. For me, it's the filling that makes this lasagna unforgettable. It is the ultimate comfort food and a meal you will want to make on repeat.

Makes 6 servings

4 tbsp (60 ml) extra virgin olive oil, divided

10 oz (283 g) baby spinach

9 oz (250 g) ricotta cheese

1 egg

½ red onion, finely chopped

3 cups (210 g) portobello mushrooms, sliced

2 cloves garlic, finely chopped

¼ lb (113 g) ground pork

¼ lb (113 g) ground beef

1 tsp oregano

½ tsp chili flakes

½ tsp cumin

¼ tsp turmeric

¼ tsp cinnamon

Sea salt and pepper

2 cups (480 ml) tomato sauce

3 tbsp (8 g) chopped fresh basil

2 (12-oz [340-g]) packages hearts of palm lasagna sheets, drained and rinsed (I used Palmini brand; see Nedi's Tips)

1 cup (110 g) shredded Manchego cheese

Preheat the oven to 400°F (205°C).

Add 2 tablespoons (30 ml) of the olive oil to a large skillet over medium heat and cook the spinach until it wilts. Let it cool and drain any liquid it may have released. Transfer the cooled spinach to a medium bowl and add the ricotta and egg. Mix well and set aside.

Meanwhile, add the remaining 2 tablespoons (30 ml) of the olive oil to the same skillet over medium heat. Toss in the onion and mushrooms and cook for 2 to 3 minutes. Add the garlic, ground pork, ground beef, oregano, chili flakes, cumin, turmeric, cinnamon, salt and pepper. Stir using a wooden spoon to break up the meat and cook for about 5 minutes, until the meat is browned.

Add the tomato sauce and reduce the heat to low. Simmer for 10 minutes and add the basil at the end.

Pour ¼ cup (60 ml) of the meat sauce into a 9 x 9–inch (23 x 23–cm) baking dish. Top with eight lasagna sheets so they cover the pan. Spread about one-third of the ricotta mix over the lasagna sheets and top with about one-third of the remaining meat sauce. Repeat these steps twice.

Sprinkle the last layer of meat sauce with the shredded cheese and bake for 15 minutes. Then, broil for 2 to 3 minutes, until golden.

Let the lasagna cool for 10 minutes before serving.

Nedi's Tips: *I buy Palmini hearts of palm lasagna sheets on Amazon; you may also be able to find them in your local health food store.*

I personally try to cook mainly with sheep or goat's milk products as they are easier to digest than cow's milk dairy. In this recipe, I used shredded Manchego to top the lasagna but the ricotta is from cow's milk. If you have an intolerance to cow's milk, a plant-based ricotta works very well as a substitution.

Tender Slow-Cooked Beef in Red Wine Tomato Sauce

This rich and hearty dish is perfect for a cold winter's day! Slow-cooked beef with vegetables and potatoes is a meal for the whole family to enjoy. If you are following a low-carb diet, try replacing the baby potatoes with artichoke bottoms. They are similar in taste and packed with more nutrients. Serve the tender slow-cooked beef with Low-Carb Potato–Cauliflower Mash (page 141) and enjoy!

Makes 8 servings

2 lb (907 g) beef chuck, cut into 2-inch (5-cm) cubes

Sea salt and pepper

4 tbsp (60 ml) extra virgin olive oil, divided

1 medium onion, diced

3 medium carrots, diced

3 celery ribs, diced

6 cloves garlic, diced

1 (14-oz [400-g]) can crushed tomatoes

½ tsp turmeric

1 tsp pepper

1 tsp coconut sugar

2 cups (480 ml) dry red wine

2 cups (480 ml) low-sodium vegetable broth

8–10 baby potatoes, cut in half

2 sprigs thyme, divided

2 bay leaves

2 tbsp (28 g) butter

2 cups (170 g) mixed mushrooms such as cremini, oyster and shiitake, sliced

1 clove garlic, minced

3 tbsp (12 g) chopped fresh parsley, for serving

Low-Carb Potato–Cauliflower Mash (page 141), for serving

Pat dry the beef with a paper towel and season it with salt and pepper. Heat 2 tablespoons (30 ml) of the olive oil in a large cast-iron pot (or Dutch oven) over medium heat and sauté the beef until it's brown on all sides. Transfer the beef to a plate and set aside.

Add the remaining 2 tablespoons (30 ml) of olive oil in the same pot and bring the heat to medium. Sauté the onions, carrots, celery and diced garlic for 2 minutes, stirring occasionally.

Add the crushed tomatoes, turmeric, pepper and coconut sugar. Stir and mix well. Add the meat back in and pour in the red wine and vegetable broth and bring to a boil. Add the baby potatoes, two sprigs of thyme and the bay leaves. Bring the heat to medium-low and cook, covered, for 2 hours. Lightly uncover for the last hour so the sauce can reduce and thicken.

Meanwhile prepare the mushrooms. In a large skillet, melt the butter and add the mushrooms, three sprigs of thyme and salt and pepper to taste. Sauté for 3 to 4 minutes, until soft. Add the minced garlic at the end, then turn off the heat and mix.

Add the mushrooms to the beef stew in the last 30 minutes of simmering time so all the flavors can combine. Remove the thyme sprigs and bay leaves before serving. Sprinkle the beef with fresh parsley and serve with Low-Carb Potato–Cauliflower Mash.

> **Nedi's Tip:** *This recipe can be made with chicken, pork or lamb. It can be stored in the fridge for 3 to 4 days; however, it's so tasty that I doubt it will last that long!*

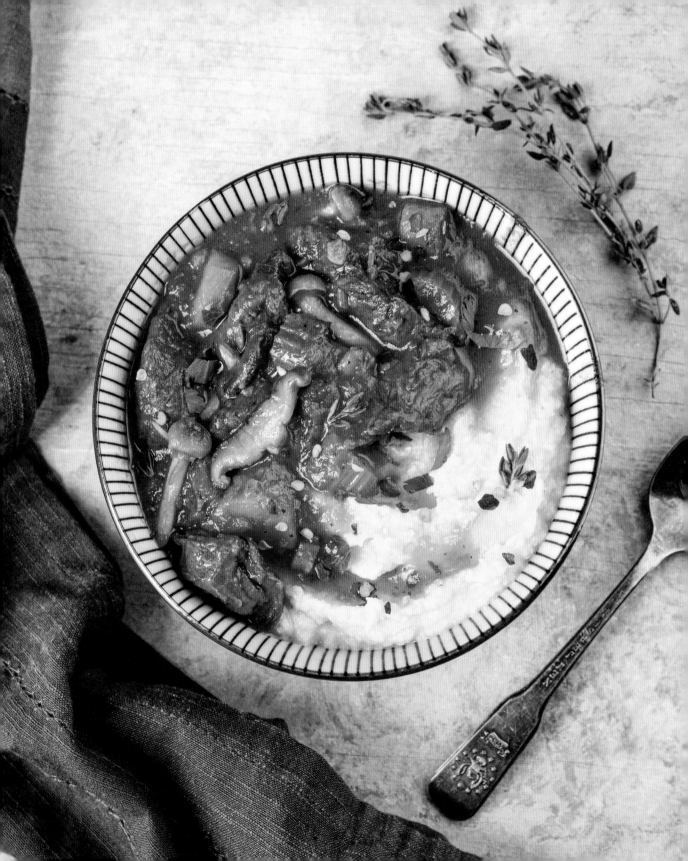

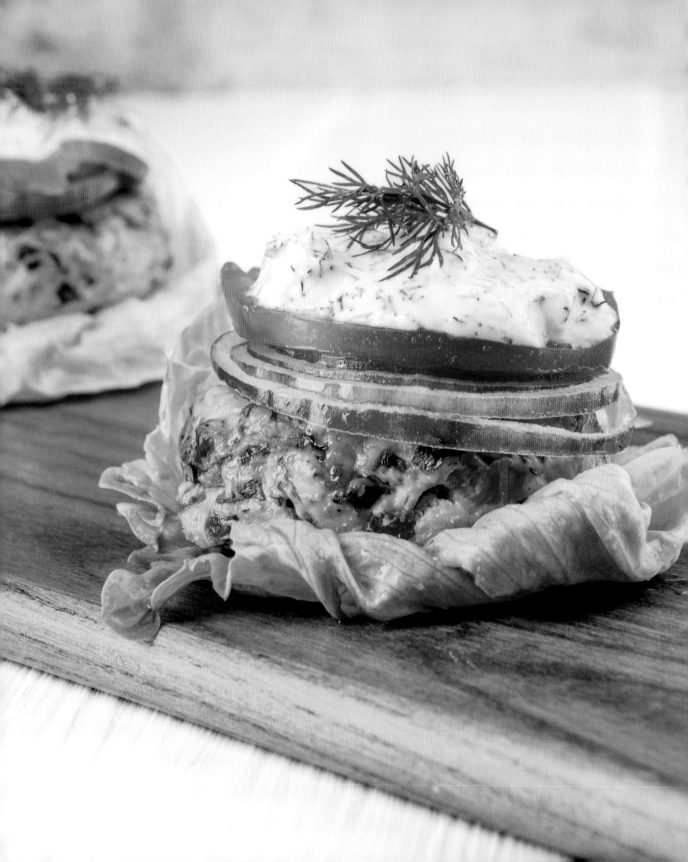

Juicy Low-Carb Turkey Burgers in Lettuce Wraps

This easy turkey burger recipe is loaded with vegetables and flavorful elements like parsley and feta cheese. The turkey patties are so juicy and tender. The burgers can be made on the grill or roasted in the oven. Both ways are equally delicious!

I love to serve the burgers in lettuce wraps for a satisfying crunch, plus it sheds some calories and carbs by removing the bun. To make this meal heartier, add a side of Red Lentil Purée (page 142).

Makes 8 patties

1 lb (454 g) lean ground turkey

1 egg

½ medium red bell pepper, finely chopped

1 jalapeño, seeds removed, finely chopped

1 cup (20 g) loosely packed arugula, finely chopped

3 green onions, finely chopped

⅓ cup (22 g) finely chopped fresh parsley

½ cup (75 g) crumbled feta cheese

½ tsp garlic powder

½ tsp sweet paprika

1 tsp oregano

Sea salt and pepper to taste

For Serving

8 leaves lettuce, such as Boston Bibb

2 tomatoes, sliced

½ red onion, thinly sliced

½ cup (120 ml) Refreshing Tzatziki (page 145)

Preheat the oven to 375°F (190°C). Line a baking tray with parchment paper.

To make the burger patties, mix the ground turkey, egg, bell pepper, jalapeño, arugula, green onions, parsley, feta, garlic powder, paprika, oregano, salt and pepper in a bowl using your hands until fully combined.

Form eight equal-sized patties and place on the parchment-lined baking sheet. Bake the patties for 20 minutes until fully cooked (being careful not to overcook them or they can become dry). Insert a food thermometer to be sure they have reached a safe temperature of 165°F (75°C).

Serve the burgers wrapped in lettuce topped with the tomatoes, red onions and Refreshing Tzatziki.

Nedi's Tip: Ground chicken works well as a substitute to the ground turkey and spinach can be used instead of the arugula.

Greek Stuffed Vegetables (Gemista)

These stuffed vegetables, known as gemista or yemista in Greek, are a popular dish made by every family throughout the Mediterranean region. The vegetables used for stuffing are usually peppers, tomatoes, zucchini and eggplant. For this recipe, I chose to use bell peppers and zucchini filled with cauliflower rice instead of traditional rice, to lighten it up. Between the vegetables, we like to add sliced potatoes to help the vegetables stay upright. The potatoes absorb all the wonderful flavors while baking in the oven and make the dish truly irresistible. This is the ultimate comfort food to impress guests and family.

Makes 8 servings

7 bell peppers (colors can be mixed)

3 zucchini

1–2 large russet potatoes, peeled and cut into wedges

Sea salt to taste

1 small onion, chopped

1 leek (white and light green part), chopped

4 cloves garlic, chopped

1 carrot, chopped

6 tbsp (90 ml) extra virgin olive oil, divided

3 cups (340 g) cauliflower rice

9 oz (250 g) ground beef

9 oz (250 g) ground pork

½ tsp cumin

½ tsp turmeric

½ tsp paprika

½ tsp chili flakes

2 tsp (4 g) dried oregano

Pepper to taste

1 large tomato, grated

¼ cup (16 g) finely chopped fresh parsley

2 tbsp (12 g) finely chopped fresh mint

1–2 cups (240–480 ml) water or vegetable broth

Refreshing Tzatziki (page 145), for serving

For the peppers, cut around the stems so the caps fall off. Remove the seeds and save the caps. For the zucchini, cut them in half crosswise and make sure the bottoms are flat so they can stand up straight. Carefully scoop out the inside of each zucchini half and set the flesh aside. Place the peppers and zucchini upright in a baking dish. Spread the potatoes around the peppers and zucchini so they don't tip over. Season the vegetables with salt.

In a food processor, place the insides of the zucchini along with the onion, leek, garlic and carrot. Pulse for a few seconds until the vegetables are finely chopped but not pureed. Heat 4 tablespoons (60 ml) of the olive oil over medium heat in a deep pot and add the vegetables from the food processor along with the cauliflower rice. Sauté the mixture for 3 to 4 minutes, stirring occasionally.

Add the ground beef and pork, cumin, turmeric, paprika, chili flakes, oregano, salt and pepper. Stir well with a wooden spoon to break up the meat so it doesn't form chunks. Cook for about 5 minutes then add the grated tomato, parsley and mint. Stir well and turn off the heat.

Preheat the oven to 400°F (205°C). Gently fill each pepper and zucchini with the vegetable and meat mixture and close the peppers with their caps. Add the water or broth to cover the peppers and zucchini halfway. Drizzle the vegetables with the remaining 2 tablespoons (30 ml) of olive oil.

Cover the pan with foil and bake for 30 minutes. After 30 minutes, remove the foil and bake for another 30 to 35 minutes, or until the potatoes are golden on top.

Transfer the vegetables to a serving platter and drizzle some of the cooking liquid on top. Serve with a side of Refreshing Tzatziki.

Nedi's Tips: You can switch the meat in this recipe up and try it out with ground chicken, lamb or veal.

For a lighter, vegan option, skip the meat and use mushrooms instead.

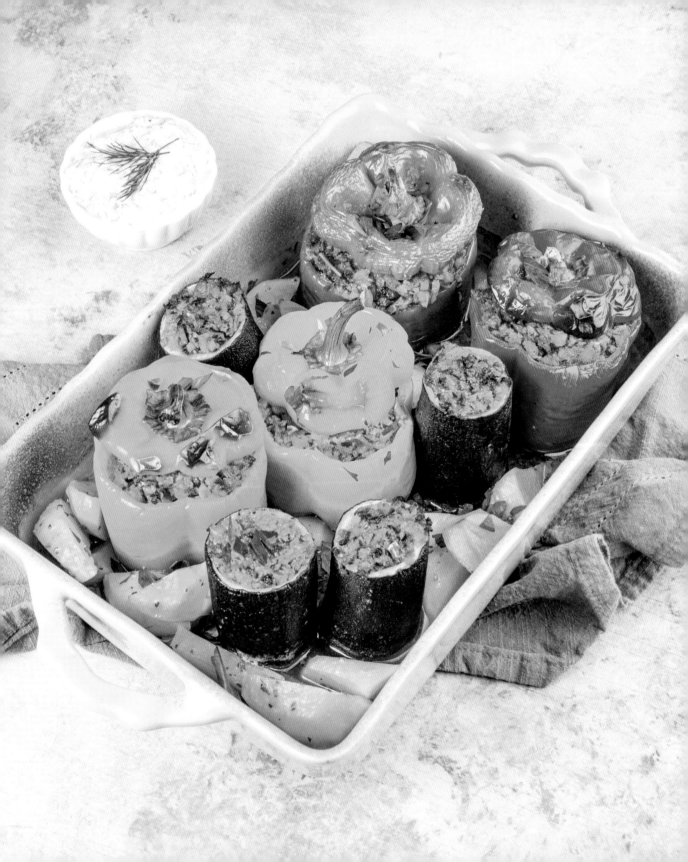

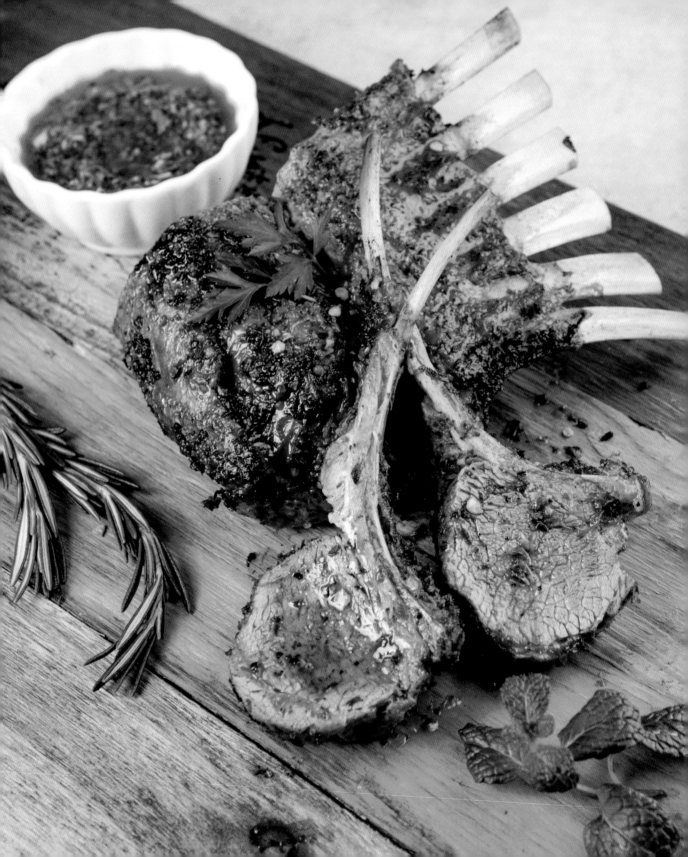

Herb-Crusted Roasted Rack of Lamb

This is an incredible roast centerpiece dish that will impress your dinner guests. It's the perfect recipe for entertaining and the holidays. The ingredients are simple and super fresh. It requires less than 10 minutes to prepare and while the lamb is roasting, you can prepare your side dishes. I love to serve the rack of lamb with Grilled Zucchini with Mint and Pine Nuts (page 138) or Refreshing Tzatziki (page 145). They complement each other so well.

Makes 4 servings

6 cloves garlic

¼ cup (60 ml) extra virgin olive oil

2 tbsp (8 g) fresh parsley

2 tbsp (11 g) fresh mint

1 tbsp (3 g) fresh rosemary

1 tbsp (5 g) dried oregano

Zest and juice from 1 lemon

1 (2-lb [907-g]) rack of lamb, Frenched

Sea salt and pepper

Preheat the oven to 450°F (230°C). Line a baking dish with parchment paper.

In a food processor, combine the garlic, olive oil, parsley, mint, rosemary, oregano, lemon zest and lemon juice. Pulse until fully pureed.

Season the lamb with salt and pepper on each side. Place the lamb rack in the parchment-lined baking dish. Spread the marinade evenly on each side of the lamb.

Roast the lamb for 15 minutes then turn over. Roast for another 10 minutes for medium–rare or 15 minutes for medium. Insert a meat thermometer; it should read 135°F (57°C) for medium rare, 145°F (63°C) for medium. Transfer the rack of lamb to a carving board and let it rest for 10 minutes before carving. Slice the lamb in between the bones and serve while warm.

> **Nedi's Tip:** *To save time, prepare the marinade ahead of time. The lamb can be marinated overnight or for a few hours in the fridge.*

Greek Meatballs (Keftedes)

These juicy Greek meatballs are incredible and always a hit at family gatherings. This is a quick and easy recipe filled with fresh herbs that is perfect for a dinner party or a quick weeknight dinner. I personally love to eat them with a Traditional Greek Salad (page 61) and Refreshing Tzatziki (page 145). Typically, when my yiayia makes these meatballs, she soaks bread and adds it to the mix, but a great low-carb trick I learned from my mom is to add Greek yogurt with a bit of baking soda to the meat mixture. It makes the meatballs juicy and fluffy.

Makes 35 meatballs

1 small red onion

1 jalapeño pepper

2 cloves garlic

3 tbsp (17 g) fresh mint

3 tbsp (12 g) fresh parsley

½ lb (226 g) ground beef

½ lb (226 g) ground pork

1 tsp oregano

1½ tsp (4 g) cumin

½ tsp cayenne pepper

2 tbsp (30 ml) plain Greek yogurt

½ tsp baking soda

1 egg

1 tbsp (15 ml) extra virgin olive oil

Sea salt and pepper to taste

Preheat the oven to 350°F (175°C). Line a baking sheet with parchment paper.

Add the onion, jalapeño, garlic, mint and parsley to a small food processor. Pulse until the vegetables and herbs are finely chopped but not pureed.

In a large bowl, mix the ground beef, ground pork, chopped vegetables and herbs, oregano, cumin, cayenne pepper, yogurt, baking soda, egg and olive oil. Season with salt and pepper and mix well using your hands until all the ingredients are well combined.

Using an ice cream scoop, form roughly 35 even-sized meatballs, and place them on the parchment-lined baking sheet about 2 to 3 inches (5 to 8 cm) apart. If they don't all fit on one baking sheet you can bake them in two batches. Bake the meatballs for 14 to 16 minutes, until brown and cooked through.

Serve the keftedes while hot and enjoy!

> **Nedi's Tip:** *My family usually pan-sears the meatballs, but to cut down on the calories and fat from the oil, I prefer to bake them. Both ways are super tasty!*

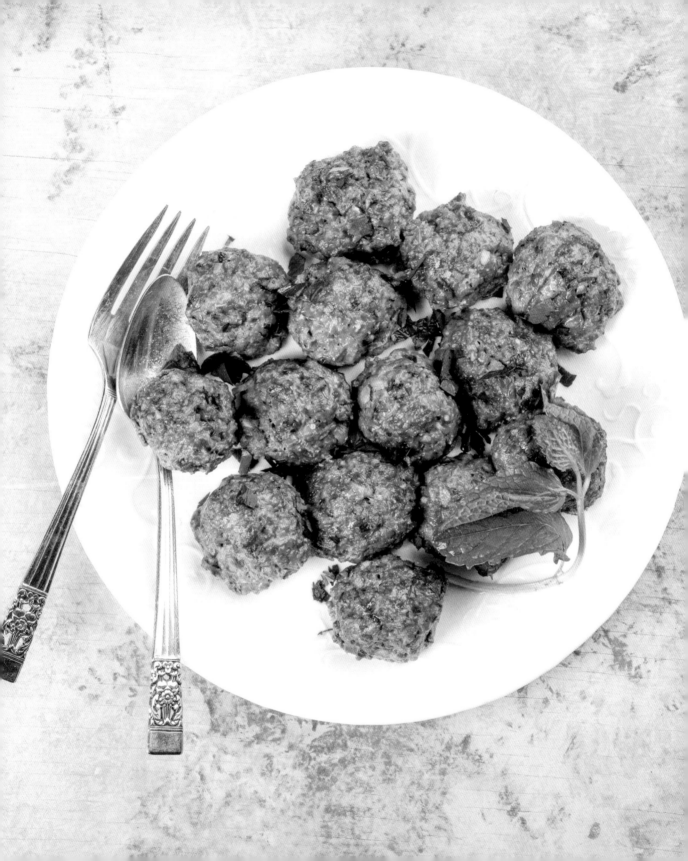

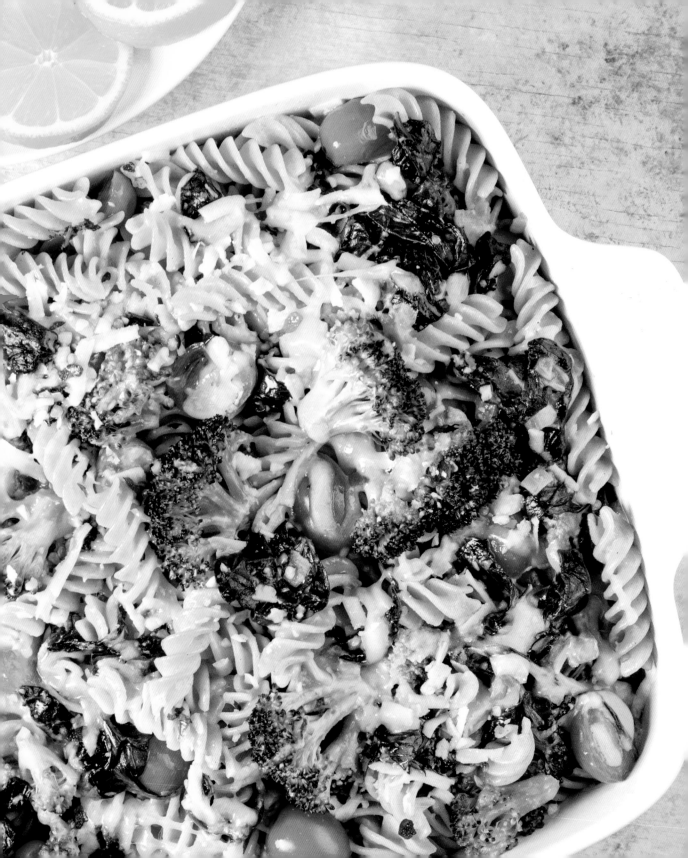

Plant-Based Mediterranean Mains

Veggies, especially when bought fresh from the farmers' market, are full of antioxidants, vitamins and minerals that will keep you feeling and looking your best. Choose seasonal, local and organic produce when possible. The dishes in this section, including Spaghetti Squash with Lentil Bolognese (page 112) and Greek Butter Beans with Spinach and Feta (page 127), are satisfying entrées that are perfect for vegetarians, vegans or anyone looking to enjoy a plant-based meal. I used vegan versions of milk and cheese in several of these dishes to keep them plant-based; if you prefer and can tolerate dairy, feel free to use your choice of cheese or milk.

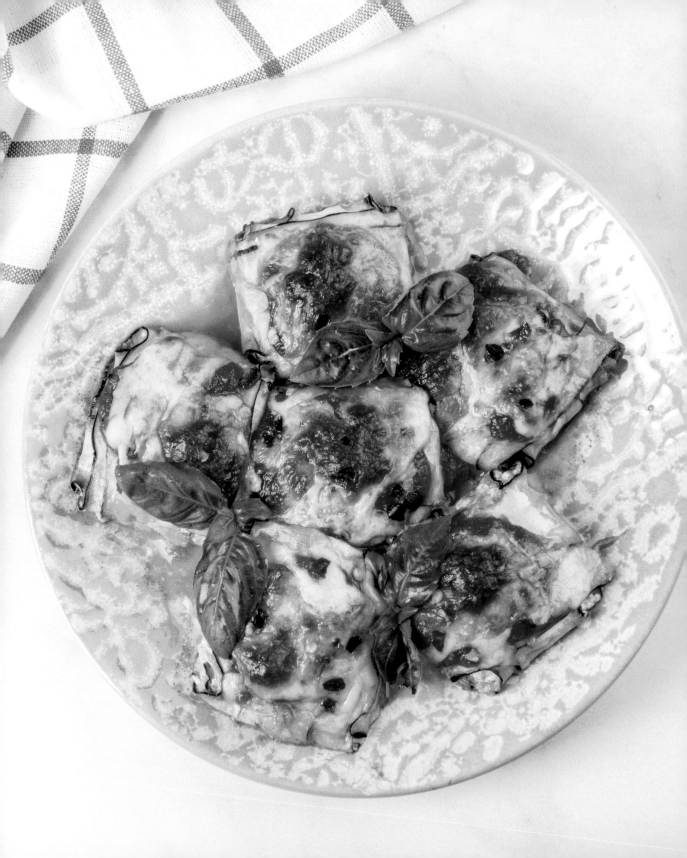

Zucchini Ravioli

These zucchini ravioli are light and filling. They will impress your taste buds and make you feel like you are dining in Italy. Packed with delicious Italian flavors of ricotta, basil and garlic, they will become one of your favorite dishes! I absolutely love how zucchini can stand in for much more than zucchini noodles. In addition to ravioli, you can get creative by making lasagna, roll-ups and even brownies using zucchini!

Makes 4 servings

3 large zucchini

1 lb (454 g) ricotta cheese

¼ cup (10 g) thinly sliced fresh basil

2 cloves garlic, minced

1 tsp oregano

1 egg

Sea salt and pepper to taste

1 cup (240 ml) tomato sauce

½ cup (56 g) shredded mozzarella

¼ tsp chili flakes

Preheat the oven to 350°F (175°C).

Cut the ends off the zucchini and, using a vegetable peeler, peel off slices of the zucchini lengthwise. Make sure the slices are very thin. I like to place paper towels between each layer of the zucchini so it can absorb excess water. Discard the thin end pieces.

In a mixing bowl, combine the ricotta, basil, garlic, oregano, egg, salt and pepper. Mix well with a fork. Transfer the zucchini to a cutting board and layer two overlapped strips vertically and two horizontally to make a cross. Repeat with the remaining slices.

Using an ice-cream scoop or spoon, scoop about 1 tablespoon (15 g) of the ricotta mixture and place it in the middle of each zucchini cross. Fold each side to seal the ricotta mixture and flip over the ravioli so the seam side is on the bottom.

In a baking dish, add a few tablespoons of tomato sauce and spread it out to cover the pan. Place the ravioli over the tomato sauce and top each ravioli with a tablespoon of the remaining sauce. Sprinkle with the shredded mozzarella. Bake for 20 to 25 minutes, until the cheese melts and is golden.

> Nedi's Tip: *To make this recipe vegan, use a vegan ricotta cheese, replace the egg with 3 to 4 tablespoons (45 to 60 ml) of nut milk and top with shredded vegan mozzarella.*

Spaghetti Squash with Lentil Bolognese

This lentil Bolognese sauce is packed with nutritious ingredients such as onion, garlic, carrots, mushrooms and lentils. The meatless sauce is tasty, hearty and meaty enough that a meat lover won't complain that anything seems missing. Spaghetti squash is a nutritious winter vegetable that offers lots of fiber, beta carotene and folate. This dish can be enjoyed with my Crunchy Green Salad with Honey-Mustard Dressing (page 54).

Makes 4 servings

1 large spaghetti squash

Sea salt and pepper, to taste

4 tbsp (60 ml) extra virgin olive oil, divided

1 medium white onion, finely chopped

1 carrot, finely chopped

3 cloves garlic, minced

2 cups (140 g) cremini mushrooms, chopped

1 (14-oz [397-g]) can cooked lentils, drained and rinsed

1 (14-oz [397-g]) can fire-roasted diced tomatoes

1 cup (240 ml) tomato sauce

2 tsp (8 g) coconut sugar

1 tsp dried oregano

1 tsp dried basil

¼ tsp chili flakes

¼ cup (10 g) chopped fresh basil, plus more for garnish

½ cup (56 g) shredded plant-based mozzarella (I used Daiya)

Preheat the oven to 400°F (205°C).

Cut the spaghetti squash in half, lengthwise, and scoop out the seeds. Season with a light pinch of salt and pepper, and drizzle with 2 tablespoons (30 ml) of the olive oil. Place the halves cut-side down on a large, rimmed baking sheet, and bake for 40 to 50 minutes, until tender. (Smaller squash will be done sooner than larger squash.) Set the squash aside to cool. When cool enough to handle, use two forks to break up the squash into noodles and place the noodles on a serving plate.

Meanwhile, make the lentil Bolognese. Heat the remaining 2 tablespoons (30 ml) of olive oil in a skillet over medium heat. Sauté the onion, carrot and garlic for 4 minutes, stirring occasionally. Add the mushrooms and sauté until they begin to soften. Add the lentils, tomatoes and tomato sauce. Stir to combine.

Stir in the coconut sugar, oregano, basil and chili flakes. Simmer the sauce for 15 minutes, until it thickens, and all the vegetables are tender. Season to taste with salt and pepper. Turn the heat off and add the fresh basil. Stir and set aside.

Spoon the lentil Bolognese over the spaghetti squash noodles and sprinkle with the mozzarella cheese. Garnish with more fresh basil and enjoy.

> **Nedi's Tip:** *Try this lentil Bolognese over zucchini noodles, gluten-free spaghetti or in a lasagna.*

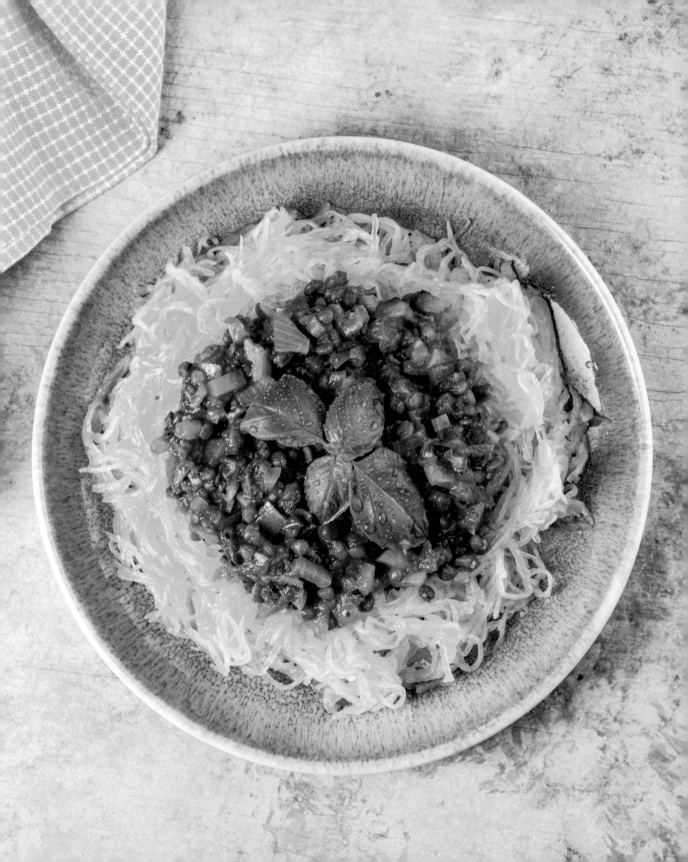

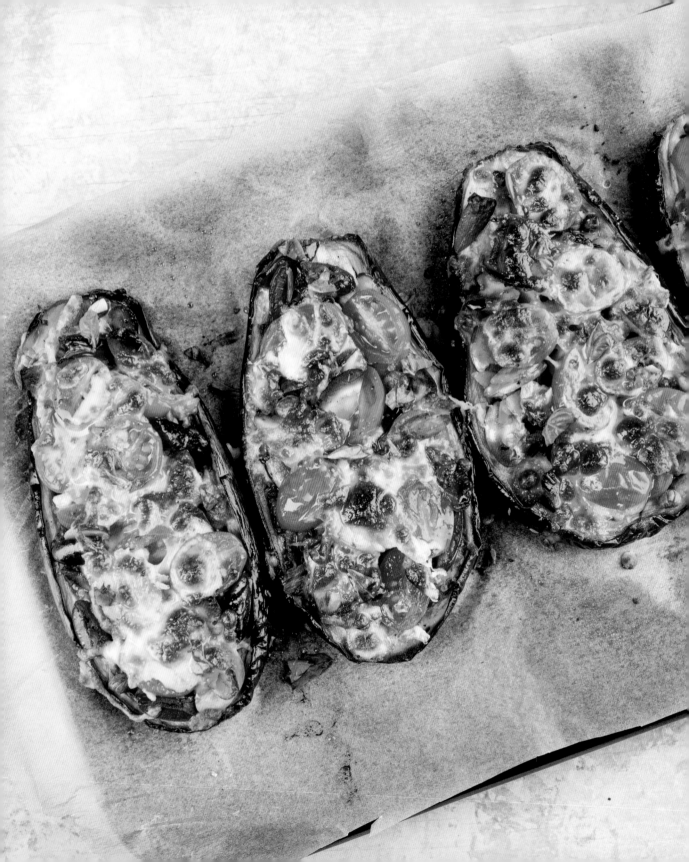

Oven-Baked Eggplant with Olives, Capers and Cheese

This rich, flavorsome baked dish is so easy to make. The Mediterranean flavors of tomatoes, olives, capers, garlic and basil will instantly make you feel like you are in a charming restaurant tucked away on the Amalfi coast.

Due to its high antioxidant content, studies have shown that incorporating eggplant into your diet may reduce the risk of heart disease. Serve this eggplant dish with a side of my Traditional Greek Salad (page 61).

Makes 4 servings

2 medium eggplants, sliced in half

Sea salt and pepper to taste

1½ cups (245 g) grape tomatoes, sliced in half

⅓ cup (40 g) Kalamata olives, pitted and chopped

½ cup (50 g) sliced raw almonds

1 tbsp (8 g) capers, chopped

2 cloves garlic, minced

2 tbsp (5 g) chopped fresh basil

1 tbsp (15 ml) extra virgin olive oil

1 tbsp (15 ml) balsamic vinegar

⅓ cup (30 g) shredded plant-based mozzarella

Preheat the oven to 400°F (205°C). Line a baking dish with parchment paper.

Arrange the eggplants in the parchment-lined baking dish. Spray the flesh sides with olive oil cooking spray and season with salt and pepper. Bake for 30 minutes, until the flesh is soft.

Remove the eggplant from the oven. Using two forks, fork the flesh of each eggplant (just like you would with spaghetti squash) and push it to the sides of the eggplant to make space in the middle for the tomato stuffing.

In a small bowl, mix the tomatoes, olives, almonds, capers, garlic, basil, olive oil and balsamic vinegar.

Fill each eggplant boat with the tomato mix and top with the grated cheese. Return to the oven for 10 to 12 minutes, until golden brown. Remove from the oven and let the eggplants cool briefly before serving.

> Nedi's Tip: *To make this a heartier meal, add ½ cup (130 g) of canned cannellini beans to the tomato mix.*

Low-Carb Eggplant Moussaka

Traditional moussaka is absolutely delicious and so comforting. It was one of my favorite meals as a child. This is my modern version of moussaka with a healthy twist. The béchamel sauce usually used in moussaka can be quite heavy; after you taste this version, you won't even miss it. This moussaka is low in carbs and high in protein, making it the perfect meal for someone who is watching their figure. The tempeh ragu tastes just like minced beef and you won't believe you are not eating meat. The moussaka pairs well with my Refreshing Tzatziki (page 145).

Makes 8 servings

4 cups (960 ml) water

1 tbsp (16 g) sea salt, plus more for sprinkling

3 medium eggplants

2 tbsp (30 ml) extra virgin olive oil

½ red onion, chopped

4 cloves garlic, chopped

1 jalapeño, seeds removed and chopped

2 cups (175 g) baby portobello mushrooms, chopped

6 oz (170 g) tempeh, finely chopped

½ tsp cumin

½ tsp cinnamon

1 tsp oregano

Sea salt and pepper to taste

2 cups (480 ml) tomato sauce

¼ cup (16 g) chopped fresh parsley

1 tbsp (12 g) coconut sugar

½ cup (56 g) shredded plant-based mozzarella (I used Daiya)

Refreshing Tzatziki (page 145), for garnish

Preheat the oven to 400°F (205°C). Line a baking sheet with parchment paper and lightly spray with cooking spray. Fill a large mixing bowl with the water and sea salt.

Slice the eggplant into ¼-inch (6-mm) circles. Place the eggplant slices in the water in the mixing bowl. This will prevent browning while you finish slicing them.

Dry the eggplant with paper towels and place the eggplant on top of the parchment-lined baking sheet. Spray the eggplant slices with a little more cooking spray and sprinkle with a little sea salt. Roast for 25 minutes. Set the eggplant aside and leave the oven on.

Heat the olive oil in a large skillet over medium heat and cook the onion for 2 to 3 minutes, until translucent. Add the garlic, jalapeño and mushrooms. Cook for another 2 minutes, until tender. Toss in the tempeh, cumin, cinnamon, oregano, sea salt and pepper. Sauté for 3 to 4 minutes, until the tempeh is slightly brown. Stir in the tomato sauce, parsley and coconut sugar and turn heat off after 1 minute.

Transfer the mixture to a high-speed food processor or blender. Pulse for 10 seconds, until it reaches a smooth consistency.

Line a 2-quart (1.9-L) oven-safe glass dish with the eggplant slices, starting with the larger slices. You should be able to fit eight slices in the first layer. Top each slice of eggplant with 1 to 2 tablespoons (15 to 30 g) of the puréed tempeh Bolognese mixture. Repeat this step by adding another two layers of eggplant and Bolognese. You should have enough for three layers of each ingredient total. Sprinkle the top with the vegan mozzarella and bake for 10 minutes, until the cheese melts.

Nedi's Tip: This moussaka can be made with lentils or ground beef instead of tempeh. I like using tempeh to replace the meat due to its health benefits. It is a fermented soybean, packed with probiotics, protein and fiber.

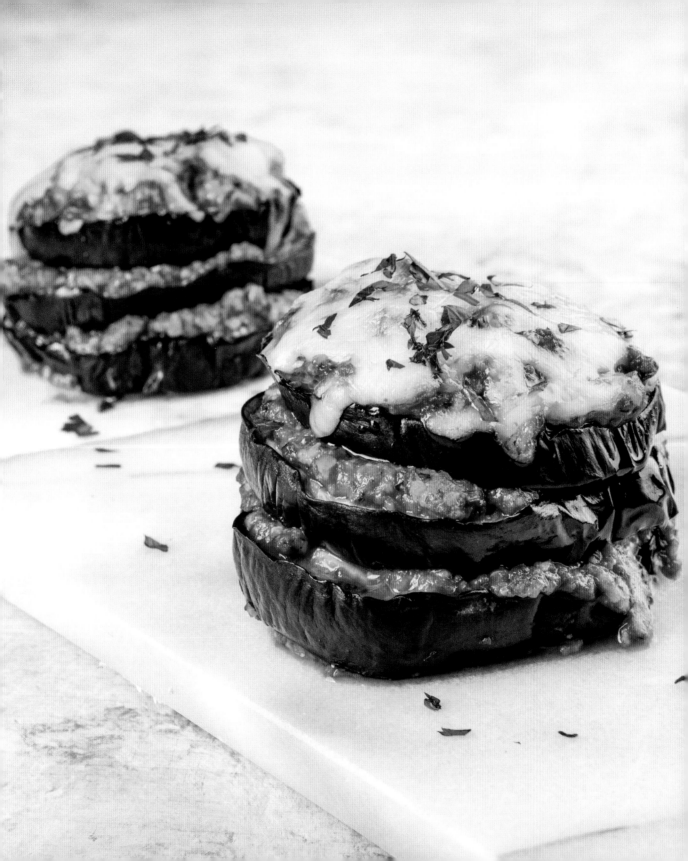

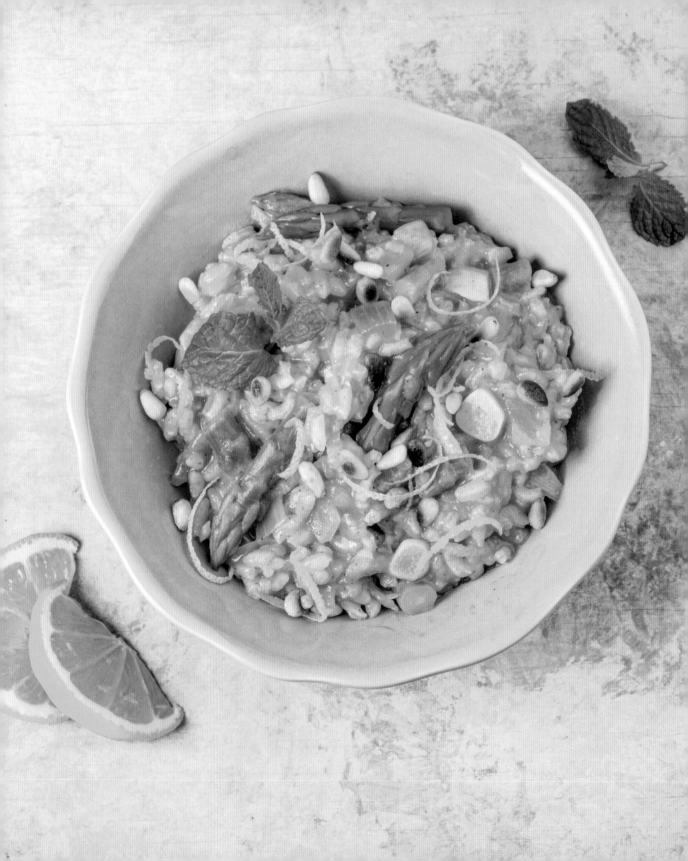

Lemon Asparagus Risotto

This vibrant risotto is perfect for a warm summer day as it isn't too heavy and is very refreshing. I love that Mediterranean cooking highlights veggies in so many dishes, and this recipe is no exception.

I decided to blend part of the asparagus with mint and basil to boost the flavor and the nutritional value of the risotto. The combination is incredible, and it will leave you going back for seconds, and probably thirds! It would make great leftovers for lunch, but when I make this recipe with my family, there are never any leftovers. I hope you enjoy it as much as we do.

Makes 4 servings

1 bunch asparagus, ends trimmed

1 cup (240 ml) warm water

¼ cup (23 g) tightly packed fresh mint, plus more for garnish (optional)

¼ cup (6 g) tightly packed fresh basil

2 tbsp (30 ml) extra virgin olive oil

½ white onion, finely diced

4 cloves garlic, minced

1 cup (180 g) Arborio rice

½ cup (120 ml) dry white wine

3½ cups (840 ml) low-sodium vegetable broth, warm

Juice and zest of 1 small lemon

¼ tsp chili flakes

Sea salt and pepper to taste

Toasted pine nuts, for garnish, optional

Rinse the asparagus and cut off the hard ends. Fill a medium pot with water and bring to a boil. Fill a large mixing bowl with water and ice.

Cook the asparagus for 2 minutes then place the asparagus spears in an ice bath to prevent overcooking and to preserve the bright green color. When the asparagus has cooled, cut it into 1-inch (2.5-cm) pieces. Fill a 1-cup (240-ml) measuring cup with the largest pieces from the bottom ends of the cooked asparagus, setting the middle pieces and the tips aside. Add the bottoms of the asparagus to a blender with the warm water, mint and basil and pulse a few times to make a creamy green sauce. Set aside.

Heat the olive oil in a large skillet over medium heat. Sauté the onion and garlic for 2 minutes. Add the rice and gently stir with a spatula, until translucent. Add the white wine and cook the risotto, stirring, until the wine evaporates.

Slowly add the warm vegetable broth, 1 cup (240 ml) at a time, stirring and allowing the rice to absorb the liquid slowly before adding more. When all the broth is absorbed, add the lemon juice, lemon zest, creamy green sauce, the rest of the asparagus, chili flakes, salt and pepper. Give it a good stir, taste and adjust seasonings to your taste. Serve the risotto topped with toasted pine nuts and mint leaves.

> **Nedi's Tips:** *To make the risotto creamier, try adding grated cheese while it's cooking.*
>
> *This risotto also tastes great topped with grilled shrimp or scallops.*

Low-Carb Zucchini Roll with Vegetables and Cheese

This zucchini roll is a delicious, low-carb, meatless dinner. Layers of sliced zucchini are filled with eggs, cheese, and a mix of sautéed vegetables then baked in the oven for an impressive gluten-free meal. It is a beautiful dish that is ideal for the holidays or a special family gathering.

Makes 8 servings

3 tbsp (45 ml) extra virgin olive oil

1 leek (white and light green part), chopped

½ red bell pepper, finely chopped

3 cups (210 g) cremini mushrooms, sliced

2 cloves garlic, chopped

1 lb (454 g) baby spinach

Sea salt and pepper to taste

2 medium zucchini, ends trimmed and thinly sliced lengthwise

4 eggs, whisked

8 thin square slices provolone cheese

1 cup (80 g) shredded pecorino cheese

1 cup (150 g) crumbled feta cheese

2 tbsp (8 g) chopped fresh parsley

8 grape tomatoes, sliced

1 cup (20 g) arugula

2 tbsp (30 ml) sriracha or a hot sauce, for drizzling

Heat the olive oil in a large skillet and sauté the leek and bell pepper for 2 to 3 minutes. Add the mushrooms and cook for 3 minutes, until they soften.

Add the garlic, spinach, salt and pepper. Sauté until the spinach is wilted. Drain any liquid it may have released and set the vegetables aside.

Preheat the oven to 400°F (205°C). Line a 9 x 13–inch (23 x 33–cm) baking dish with parchment paper and lightly spray with olive oil cooking spray.

Line the sliced zucchini in the pan so they cover the bottom completely. They may overlap and that's ok. Bake in the oven for 20 minutes, until they become soft. Remove from the oven.

Pour the whisked eggs over the zucchini and spread out evenly. Place back in the oven and cook for 5 minutes. Remove from the oven.

Top the zucchini layers with the slices of provolone cheese. Spread the cooked vegetable mix over the cheese layer. Top with the pecorino and feta. Place back into the oven for 7 minutes.

Take the pan out and let it rest for 5 minutes. Starting on one of the long sides of the pan, use the parchment paper to help you lift and slowly roll the zucchini, tucking it under as you go. Continue to tuck until it forms a roll, leaving the parchment paper in the pan so it's easier to transfer later. Place it back in the oven for 5 to 8 minutes, until it is golden on top.

Carefully transfer the roll to a serving platter. Sprinkle with the chopped parsley and decorate with sliced grape tomatoes. Spread the arugula around the dish and drizzle with the sriracha. Serve while warm and enjoy.

Nedi's Tips: *Plant-based cheese can be used if desired.*

The stuffing can be made with many different ingredients. I've used shredded chicken, which tastes divine.

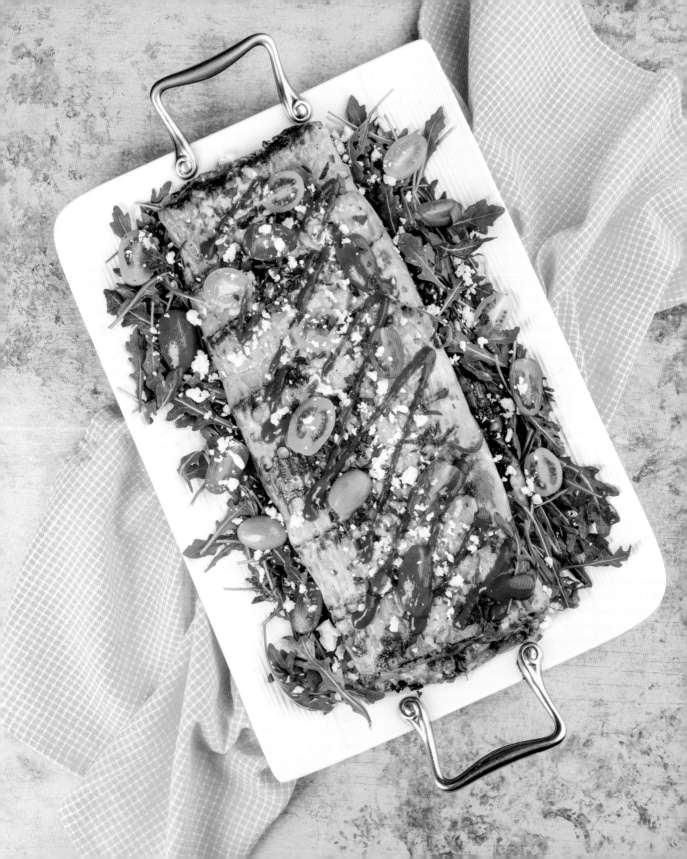

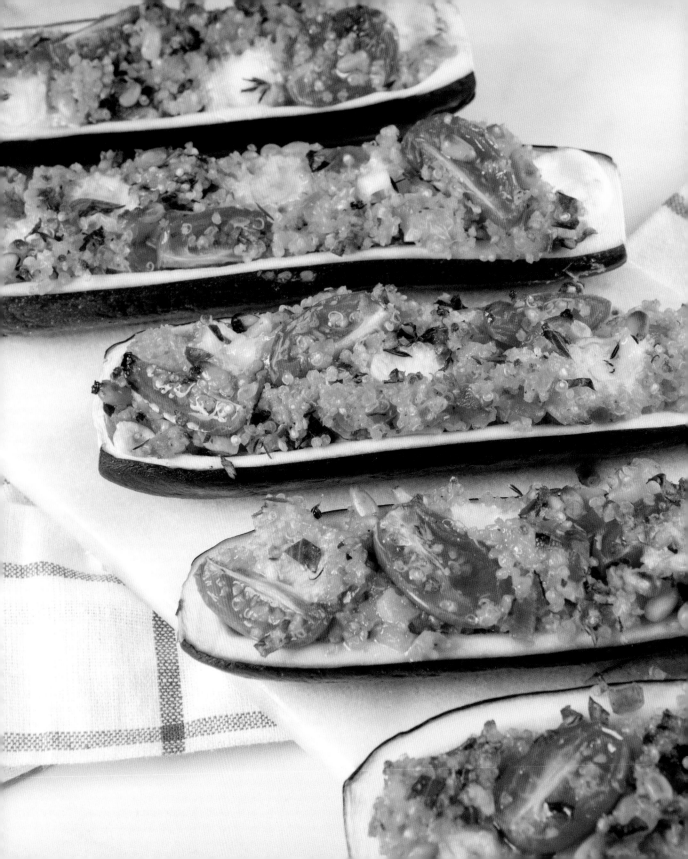

Veggie-Stuffed Zucchini Boats

Zucchini boats are a beautiful and healthy dish that will become a staple for your weeknight meals. This is an easy recipe, packed with flavor, protein and fiber. The combination of fiber and protein will keep you satiated for a while. I recommend serving the zucchini boats with a side of Arugula and Avocado Salad with Strawberry Dressing (page 57).

Makes 4 servings

⅓ cup (60 g) quinoa

4 zucchini

2 tbsp (30 ml) extra virgin olive oil

½ red onion, finely diced

3 green onions, finely chopped

3 cloves garlic, minced

½ tsp thyme

½ tsp hot paprika

¼ tsp turmeric

Sea salt and pepper to taste

½ cup (75 g) cherry tomatoes, sliced in half

3 tbsp (12 g) chopped fresh parsley

2 tbsp (8 g) chopped fresh mint

¼ cup (30 g) pine nuts

½ cup (75 g) crumbled plant-based feta

Cook the quinoa per the package directions and set aside. (See Nedi's Tips.)

Meanwhile, preheat the oven to 400°F (205°C). Cut the zucchini in half lengthwise and scoop out the center/pulp of the zucchini. Place the pulp onto a paper towel to absorb the excess liquid then dice into small pieces. Set aside.

Line a baking sheet with parchment paper and place the zucchini boats on top (skin-side down). Bake the zucchini for 15 minutes, until tender. Remove them from the oven and use a paper towel to blot up any excess liquid.

Heat the olive oil over medium heat in a large skillet. Sauté the onion, green onions, garlic and the zucchini pulp. Season with the thyme, paprika, turmeric, salt and pepper. Turn off the heat and toss in the quinoa, cherry tomatoes, parsley, mint and pine nuts. Mix well.

Spread the quinoa mixture evenly into the zucchini boats. Top each zucchini boat with some of the plant-based feta. Roast the zucchini for 12 minutes, until the cheese melts. Serve immediately or at room temperature.

> Nedi's Tips: *For extra flavor, I like to cook the quinoa in vegetable broth.*
>
> *Try adding chickpeas or lentils to up the protein.*

Creamy Chickpea Fusilli with Broccoli and Spinach

This creamy pasta comes together quickly and makes a delicious, comforting meatless meal. The chickpea fusilli are gluten free, lower in carbohydrates than traditional pasta and a rich source of fiber and protein. The veggies in this dish turn this pasta into a complete meal that will keep you feeling full for hours. Serve it with my Crunchy Green Salad with Honey-Mustard Dressing (page 54) or as a side to my Juicy Low-Carb Turkey Burgers (page 101).

Makes 6 servings

8 oz (226 g) chickpea fusilli pasta

1 head broccoli

2 tbsp (30 ml) extra virgin olive oil

1 small yellow onion, finely chopped

1 lb 2 oz (500 g) baby spinach

3 cloves garlic, finely chopped

1 cup (150 g) cherry tomatoes, sliced in half

Sea salt and pepper to taste

1 cup (240 ml) canned coconut milk

Zest and juice of ½ lemon

½ cup (40 g) mixed shredded cheese such as Manchego and pecorino Romano

3 tbsp (8 g) chopped fresh basil

¼ tsp chili flakes

Cook the chickpea fusilli pasta per package directions. Reserve ½ cup (120 ml) of the cooking water and drain the rest. Set aside.

Wash the broccoli and cut it into florets. Bring a pot of water to a boil and steam the broccoli for 5 to 7 minutes, until tender. Set aside.

Heat the olive oil in a large skillet over medium heat. Cook the onion for 2 to 3 minutes, until it becomes translucent, then add the baby spinach. Sauté while stirring occasionally until the spinach has wilted.

Add the garlic and cherry tomatoes. Season with salt and pepper to taste. Cook for 1 minute then add the coconut milk. Add the cooked fusilli and broccoli to the skillet. Turn off the heat and top with the lemon zest and lemon juice. Gently toss to combine and garnish with the shredded cheese, fresh basil and chili flakes. Add some of the reserved pasta cooking water if the consistency needs more liquid.

Preheat the oven to 375°F (190°C). Transfer the fusilli to an 8 x 8–inch (20 x 20–cm) baking dish and cover the dish with foil. Bake, covered, for 10 minutes then uncover and bake for 5 more minutes. Serve while hot and enjoy.

> Nedi's Tip: *This pasta can be made with any vegetables you have on hand. I have added zucchini, leek, and mushrooms in place of the broccoli and spinach. The warm and cheesy vegetables are what make this pasta dish a total star!*

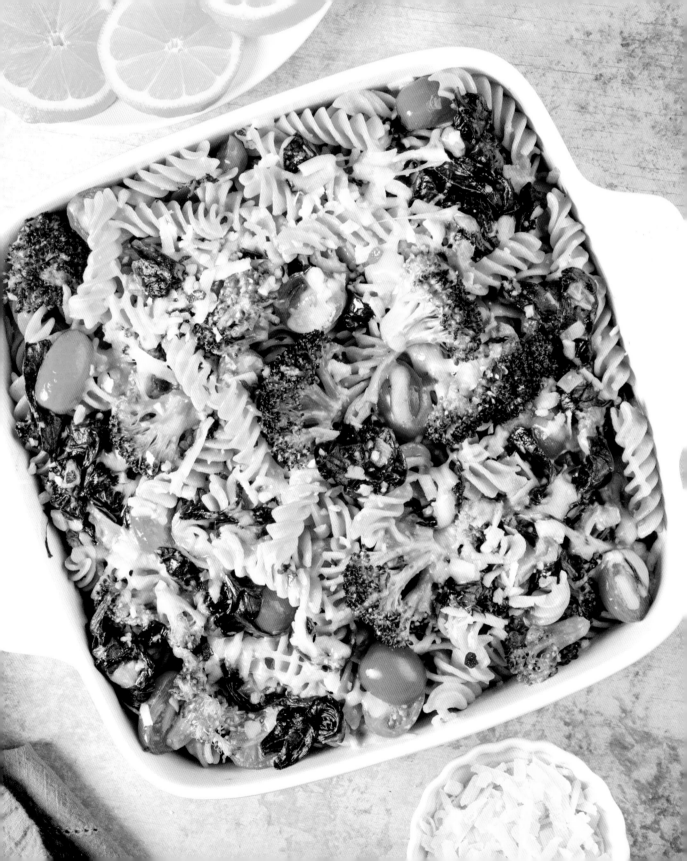

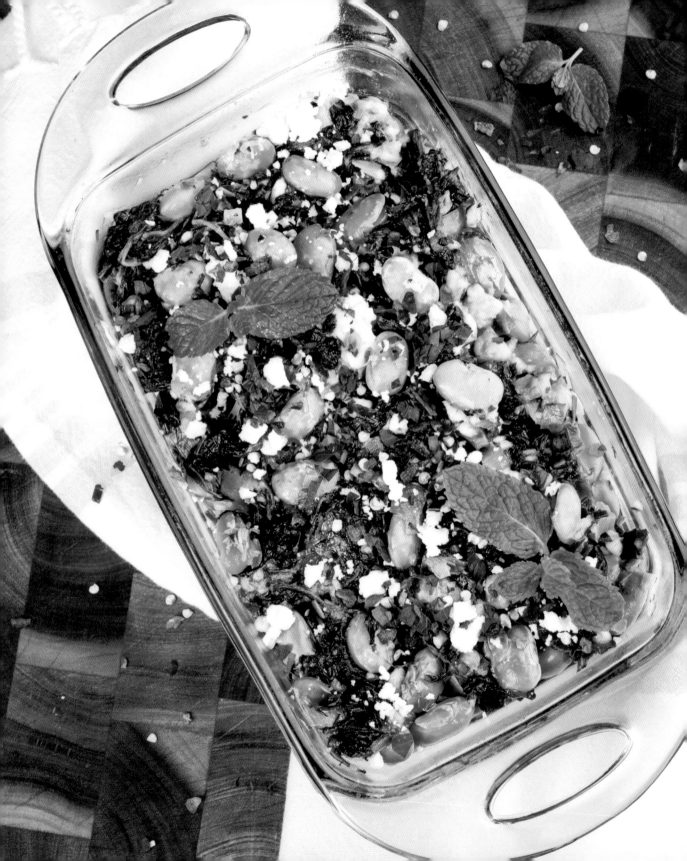

Greek Butter Beans with Spinach and Feta

This dish is known as "gigantes" in Greece, which means giants. My family typically makes this dish with a red tomato sauce. It's hearty and delicious, but I gave this family classic my own twist. The combination of spinach, leeks and feta is one of the tastiest flavors you will try. The feta can be substituted with vegan feta or another type of cheese of your choice.

Makes 8 servings

1 lb (454 g) dry white giant beans or butter beans

Pinch of sea salt, plus more to taste

3 tbsp (45 ml) extra virgin olive oil

1 red onion, finely chopped

1 leek (white and light green part), finely chopped

1 celery rib with leaves, finely chopped

5 green onions, finely chopped

1 lb 2 oz (500 g) spinach, chopped

3 tbsp (12 g) chopped fresh parsley

3 tbsp (12 g) chopped fresh mint

1 tsp oregano

¼ tsp chili flakes

Pepper to taste

2 tbsp (30 ml) fresh lemon juice

1 cup (150 g) crumbled feta cheese

Soak the beans in a large pot filled with water overnight. Drain the beans and rinse them with cold water.

Place the beans back into the pot and fill it up with water, enough to cover them. Add a pinch of sea salt and bring to a boil. Lower the heat to medium and cook for 1 hour, until the beans become soft. Drain the beans and reserve the water.

Meanwhile, heat the olive oil in a large skillet over medium heat. Sauté the onion, leek, celery and green onions for 3 to 4 minutes, until soft. Add the spinach and cook until wilted. Add the parsley, mint, oregano and chili flakes, and season with salt and pepper.

Add the cooked beans to the spinach mix and stir with a spoon. Pour in 1¼ cups (300 ml) of the reserved bean cooking water. Add the lemon juice and feta. Mix well.

Preheat the oven to 375°F (190°C). Transfer the beans to an oval baking dish and bake for 30 minutes. Serve hot or at room temperature.

Nedi's Tips: *Try adding broccoli rabe or kale instead of spinach to change up the flavors!*

You can use canned beans instead of dried to save time if you'd like. Use three 15.5-oz (439-g) cans of butter beans.

Red Lentil Spaghetti with Artichokes and Olives

This healthy Mediterranean pasta is so effortless and delicious! I love recipes like this that combine pantry staples and fresh ingredients to create a fast, healthy meal.

If you are looking for a protein-rich alternative to traditional spaghetti, red lentil spaghetti will be your new best friend. It has great texture and taste and is packed with fiber, protein, calcium and potassium. Red lentil pasta is a great substitute to regular noodles and ideal for those who are watching their carb intake.

Makes 4 servings

9 oz (250 g) red lentil spaghetti

3 tbsp (45 ml) extra virgin olive oil

4 cloves garlic, minced

1 ½ cups (225 g) cherry tomatoes, sliced in half

¼ cup (60 ml) white wine

3 tbsp (23 g) Kalamata olives, pitted and sliced in half

1 cup (168 g) canned artichoke hearts, sliced in half

3 tbsp (25 g) capers

¼ tsp chili flakes

Sea salt and pepper to taste

Zest and juice of ½ lemon

5 tbsp (20 g) chopped parsley

Grated Parmesan cheese, for garnish, optional

Bring a large pot of water to a boil and cook the spaghetti until al dente. Reserve ½ cup (120 ml) of the pasta cooking water, then drain.

Meanwhile, heat the olive oil in a large skillet over medium heat and add the garlic and cherry tomatoes. Cook for 2 to 3 minutes, until the garlic is fragrant, and the tomatoes begin to release their juices.

Add the white wine, olives, artichoke hearts and capers. Cook for 1 minute then add the cooked spaghetti. If the sauce seems too dry, add some of the reserved pasta water. Season with the chili flakes, salt and pepper. Add the lemon juice, lemon zest and parsley. Toss lightly and serve while hot. Sprinkle with Parmesan cheese if desired.

Nedi's Tips: The lentil spaghetti should be eaten right away. If you let it sit out for a while it may harden.

For additional heart-healthy protein and fats, I recommend adding canned tuna if you are not vegan or a can of chickpeas for those following a plant-based diet.

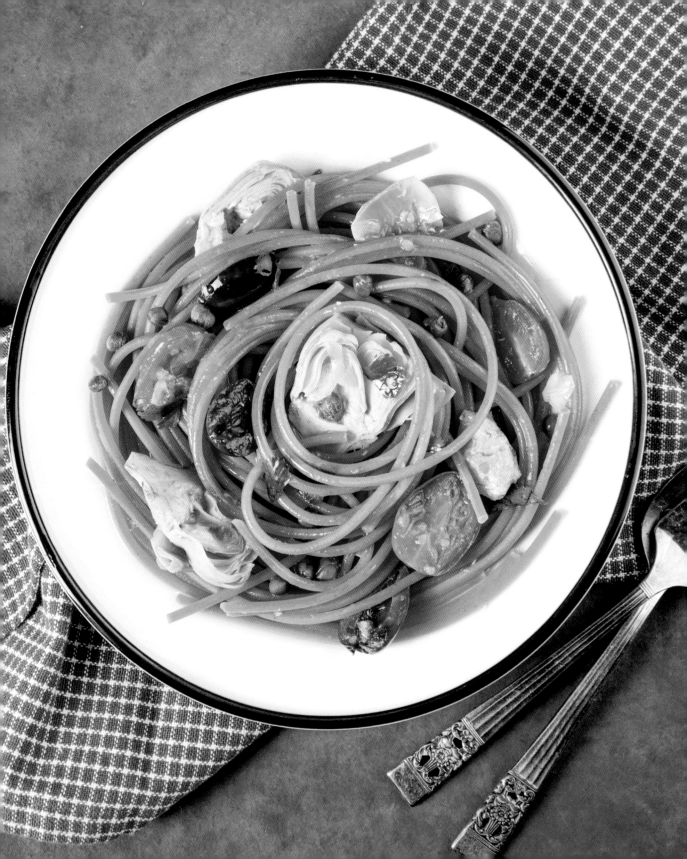

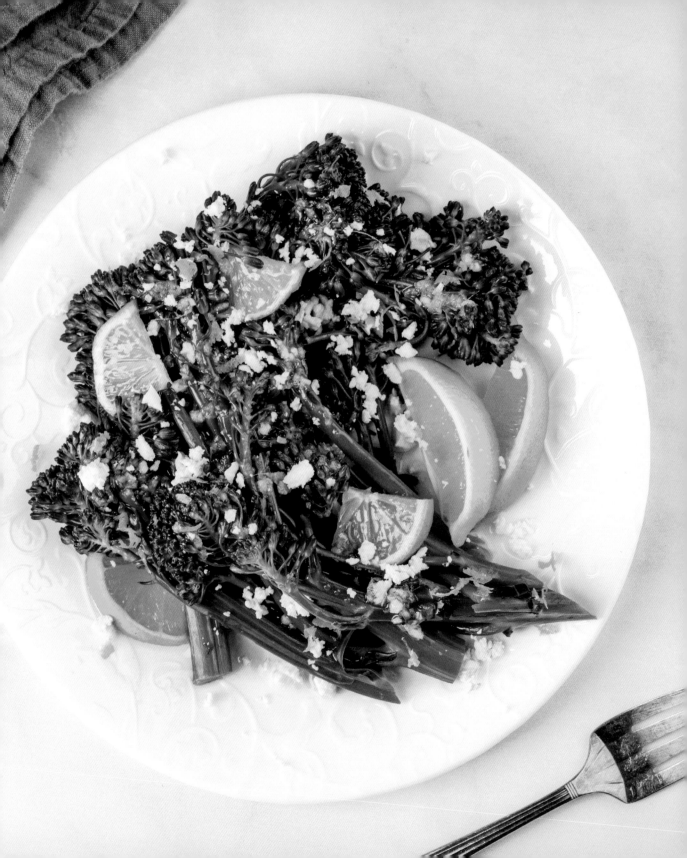

Traditional Side Dishes and Dips

Mediterranean dips are healthy, appetizing and versatile, making them useful for almost any dining event. I love entertaining guests with my Spicy Greek Feta Dip (page 149) and Roasted Red Pepper Hummus (page 146).

Mediterranean side dishes are equally delectable. With recipes such as Grilled Zucchini with Mint and Pine Nuts (page 138) and Broccolini with Garlic, Lemon Zest and Feta (page 137), these sides can not only complement a variety of many main dishes, but they are also brimming with nutrients.

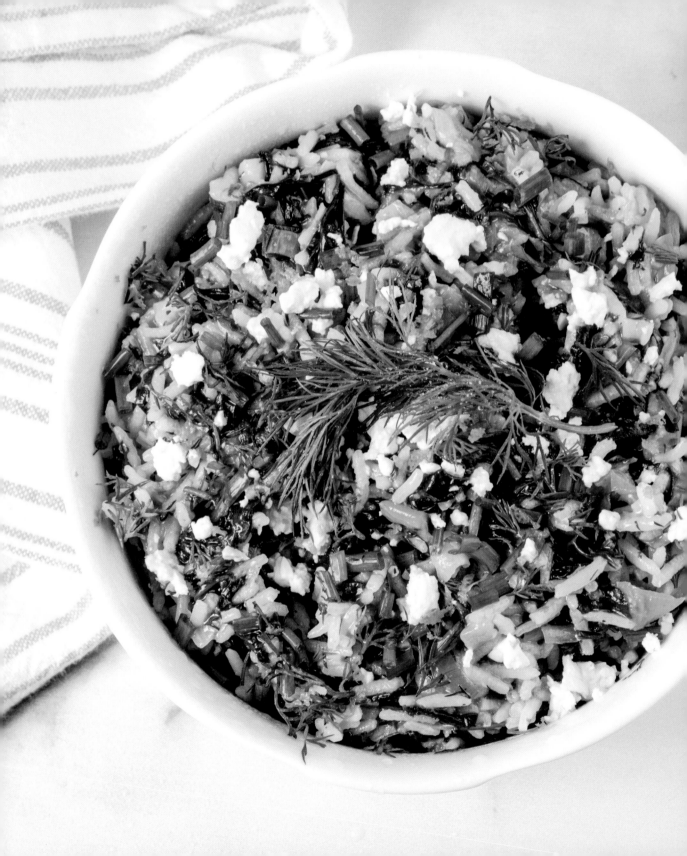

Greek Spinach Rice (Spanakorizo)

Spanakorizo is a classic vegetarian Greek dish made with a lot of spinach and fresh herbs. There are many variations to this dish. Some people like to use parsley instead of dill, while others prefer green onions versus chives. Tailor it to your taste and get creative! This simple, healthy and authentic Greek dish makes a filling meal, and it is also a great side dish to grilled meats or fish. The lemon zest, dill and chives add so much flavor and give it an extraordinary aroma.

Makes 4 servings

2 tbsp (30 ml) extra virgin olive oil

1 onion, finely chopped

1 leek (white and light green part), finely chopped

3 cloves garlic, finely chopped

¼ cup (12 g) chopped chives, divided

16 oz (454 g) baby spinach

¾ cup (150 g) white basmati rice

2 cups (480 ml) low sodium vegetable broth or water

Sea salt and pepper to taste

¼ cup (13 g) finely chopped fresh dill

Juice and zest of 1 small lemon

Chopped chives or green onions, for garnish, optional

Crumbled feta cheese, for garnish, optional

Heat the olive oil in a large pot over medium heat. Sauté the onion, leek and garlic for 2 minutes, or until translucent. Add 2 tablespoons (6 g) of the chives and the baby spinach. Cook for 3 to 4 minutes, until the spinach is wilted.

Add the basmati rice, vegetable broth, salt and pepper and stir. Bring to a boil, cover with a lid and reduce the heat to low. Simmer for 15 minutes.

Turn off the heat and stir in the fresh dill, lemon juice and lemon zest. Garnish with the remaining 2 tablespoons (6 g) of chives or green onions and feta.

Nedi's Tips: *Make sure not to overmix the rice after it is done cooking. This will prevent it from getting mushy.*

For a lighter version, try substituting the rice with cauliflower rice. You would need about 4 cups (450 g) of cauliflower rice. If you use cauliflower rice instead, you can skip the vegetable broth and water and 15-minute cook time and just sauté the cauliflower for 5 minutes after sautéing the onion, leek and garlic.

Baby Potatoes with Garlic and Dill

This recipe brings me back to my childhood. I used to love it as a kid, and I still do! It's a classic recipe my mom would often make for Easter to serve with roasted lamb. The skin of the baby potatoes is so tender, it doesn't have to be peeled. Serve this dish with Herb-Crusted Roasted Rack of Lamb (page 105) or with Oven Roasted Sea Bream (page 67).

Makes 4 servings

1 lb (454 g) honey gold baby potatoes

1 tsp sea salt

1 tbsp (14 g) butter

3 cloves garlic, finely chopped

2 tbsp (7 g) finely chopped fresh dill

Fill a medium saucepan with water and bring to a boil. Add the salt and potatoes and cook for 20 minutes or until tender. Drain the potatoes in a colander and transfer to a skillet.

Add the butter to the potatoes, and gently toss. Cook for 2 to 3 minutes and add the garlic. Turn off the heat and garnish the potatoes with the dill. Give the potatoes a good stir, cover the skillet and shake a few times so all the ingredients mix well together.

> Nedi's Tip: *Artichoke bottoms can be used in this recipe in place of potatoes. They are low carb, ranked as the number one antioxidant vegetable and are used as a digestive aid to reduce bloating and promote regularity. If you would like to try this with canned artichoke bottoms, simply sauté them lightly, then mix with the other ingredients. Frozen artichoke bottoms can also be used but may take more time to cook.*

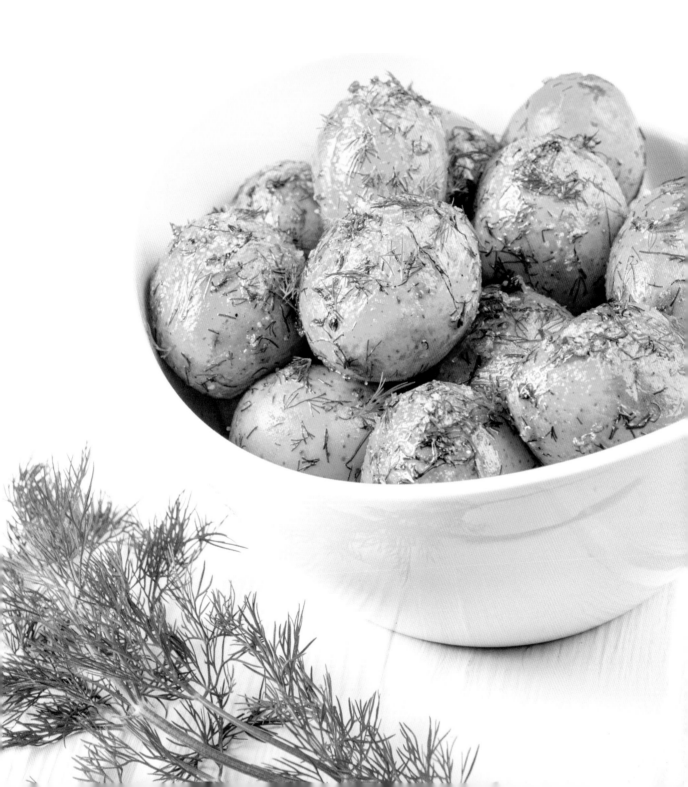

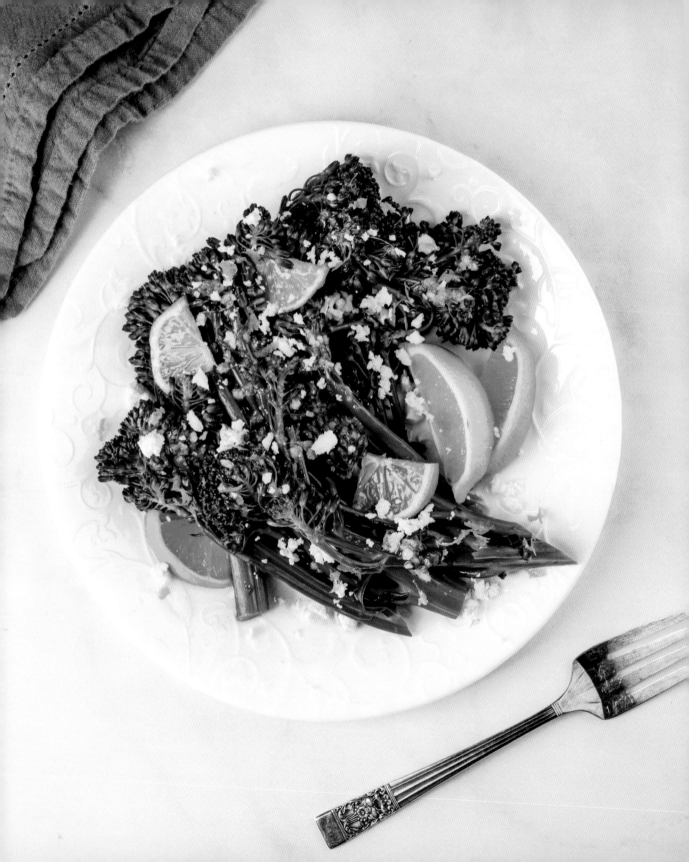

Broccolini with Garlic, Lemon Zest and Feta

This is one of those side dishes that goes well with just about anything. It is so easy to prepare, and the dressing adds a great flavor. My yiayia knows how much I love greens, and often makes this recipe for me. She usually uses broccoli so if you can't find broccolini in the grocery store, a head of broccoli will work just as well.

Makes 4 servings

2 bunches broccolini, ends trimmed and peeled

½ lemon, juiced and zested, separated

1 clove garlic, minced

1 tbsp (15 g) grated fresh ginger

3 tbsp (45 ml) extra virgin olive oil

Sea salt and pepper to taste

2 tbsp (15 g) crumbled feta cheese, for serving

Fill a pot with water and bring to a boil. Add the broccolini and cook for 7 to 8 minutes, covered. Meanwhile, fill a large bowl with water and ice and set it next to the stove. After 7 to 8 minutes, test the broccolini with a fork to see if it's tender. If not, cook an extra minute but don't cook it for more than 10 minutes. Using tongs or a slotted spoon, transfer the broccolini to the prepared ice bath to keep it from overcooking. Drain, then transfer to a serving plate.

In a small bowl, combine the lemon juice, garlic, ginger, olive oil, salt and pepper. Mix well and drizzle over the broccolini. Toss and serve with the lemon zest and feta.

> *Nedi's Tip: This side can be made ahead of time and stored in the fridge for 2 days.*

Grilled Zucchini with Mint and Pine Nuts

This is a simple and healthy side dish that is easy to whip up within 10 minutes. It is perfect for any grilled meat, fish or chicken. Toasting the pine nuts brings out an earthy flavor and makes the zucchini taste incredible.

Makes 4 servings

3 medium zucchini, ends trimmed and sliced lengthwise

3 tbsp (45 ml) extra virgin olive oil

Sea salt and pepper to taste

3 tbsp (23 g) pine nuts, toasted

3 tbsp (12 g) chopped fresh mint

Juice of 1 lime

¼ tsp chili flakes

2 tbsp (14 g) crumbled goat cheese, for garnish, optional

Preheat a grill or grill pan over medium heat. Brush the zucchini with the olive oil and season with salt and pepper. Grill for 3 to 4 minutes per side, until tender.

Place the pine nuts in a small, dry, nonstick skillet and heat over medium heat. Cook for 2 to 3, tossing occasionally so they don't burn. As soon as they start turning golden, remove from the heat.

Top the zucchini with the pine nuts, fresh mint, lime juice and chili flakes. Enjoy this dish warm or cold. If you'd like, sprinkle with crumbled goat cheese.

Nedi's Tip: *Lightly drizzle the zucchini with a balsamic glaze for extra flavor.*

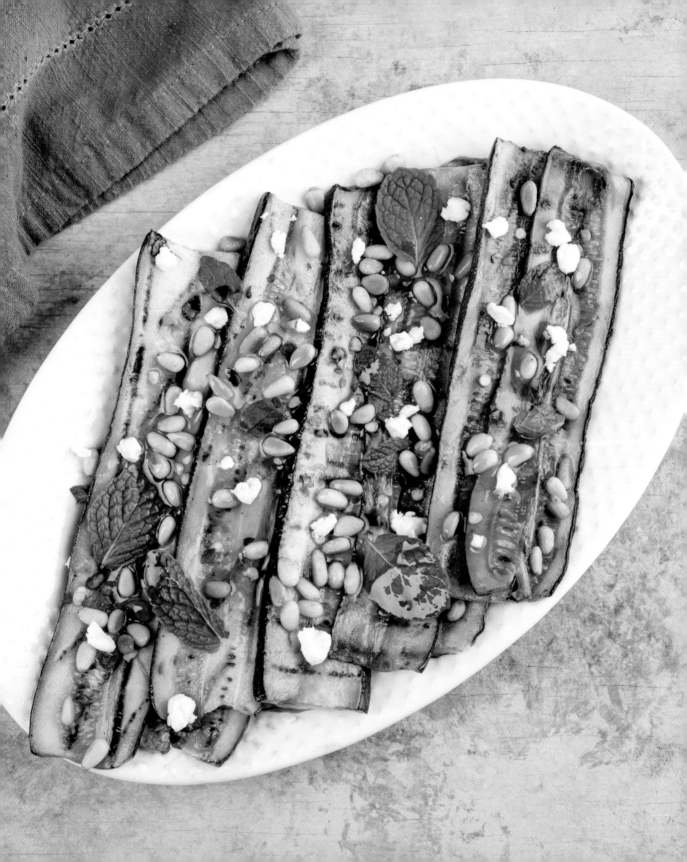

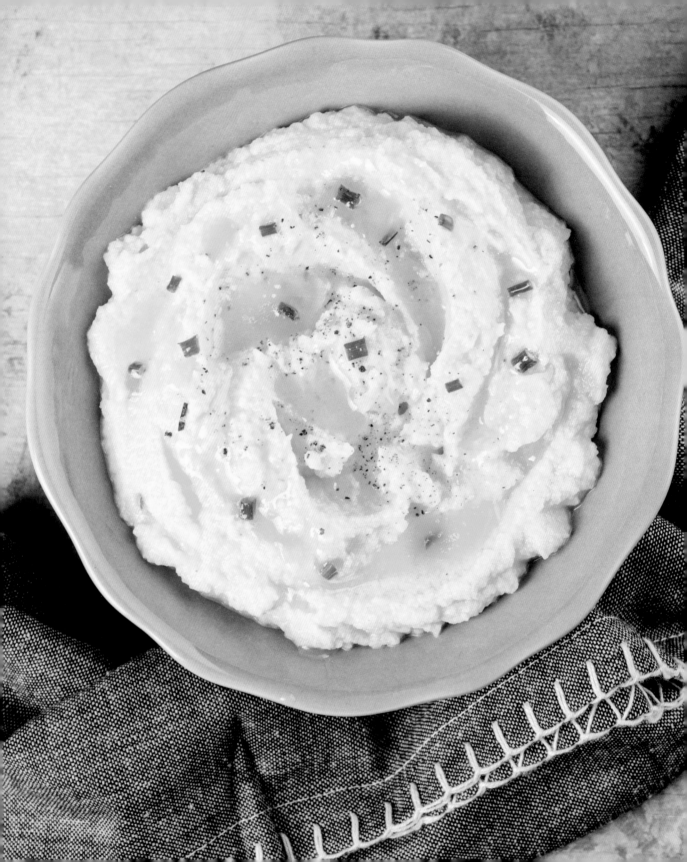

Low-Carb Potato-Cauliflower Mash

This cauliflower mash will easily become your new favorite side dish! It is lighter than regular mashed potatoes because of the cauliflower. I love the combination of cauliflower and potato as a purée. They pair so well together, and you get to sneak in extra nutrients and vitamins without compromising the taste.

Makes 6 servings

1 medium head cauliflower, chopped

1 medium potato, skin on and chopped

3 tbsp (45 ml) plain Greek yogurt

1 tbsp (14 g) butter

¼ tsp turmeric

Sea salt and pepper to taste

2 tbsp (6 g) finely chopped chives, for serving

Fill a pot with water and bring to a boil. Add the cauliflower and potato and cook until tender, about 20 minutes. Drain well.

Add the cauliflower, potato, yogurt, butter, turmeric, salt and pepper to a food processor. Pulse for 20 to 30 seconds, until it forms a purée consistency. Transfer to a serving bowl, garnish with chives and a little bit of fresh cracked pepper.

> **Nedi's Tip:** *This recipe can be made vegan using a dairy-free yogurt and olive oil in place of Greek yogurt and butter.*

Red Lentil Purée

This red lentil purée is flavorful and nutrient packed. Lentils are low in calories, rich in iron and an excellent source of fiber and protein. Red lentils cook quickly and become very soft, making it a great side dish for a homey weeknight dinner. This purée tastes incredible as a side to Oven Roasted Sea Bream (page 67).

Makes 4 servings

1 cup (192 g) red lentils

1 carrot, chopped

1 small yellow onion, chopped

1 qt (960 ml) water

1 tbsp (15 ml) extra virgin olive oil, plus more for drizzling

1 tbsp (15 ml) fresh lemon juice

2 tbsp (8 g) fresh parsley, plus more for garnish

2 cloves garlic

1 tsp sea salt

1 tsp oregano

½ tsp cumin

½ tsp chili flakes

Place the red lentils, carrot and onion in a small pot and add the water. Bring to a boil, uncovered, then lower the heat. Cook for 15 minutes. Drain the cooked lentils and transfer to a food processor.

Add the olive oil, lemon juice, parsley, garlic, salt, oregano, cumin and chili flakes to the food processor. Pulse until the mixture becomes smooth. Transfer to a serving bowl and drizzle with a little bit of olive oil and garnish with chopped parsley. This dish can be eaten hot or at room temperature.

> Nedi's Tip: *This purée freezes well and can be stored in the freezer for up to 6 months. When ready to eat, defrost overnight in the fridge and heat it up in a small pot.*

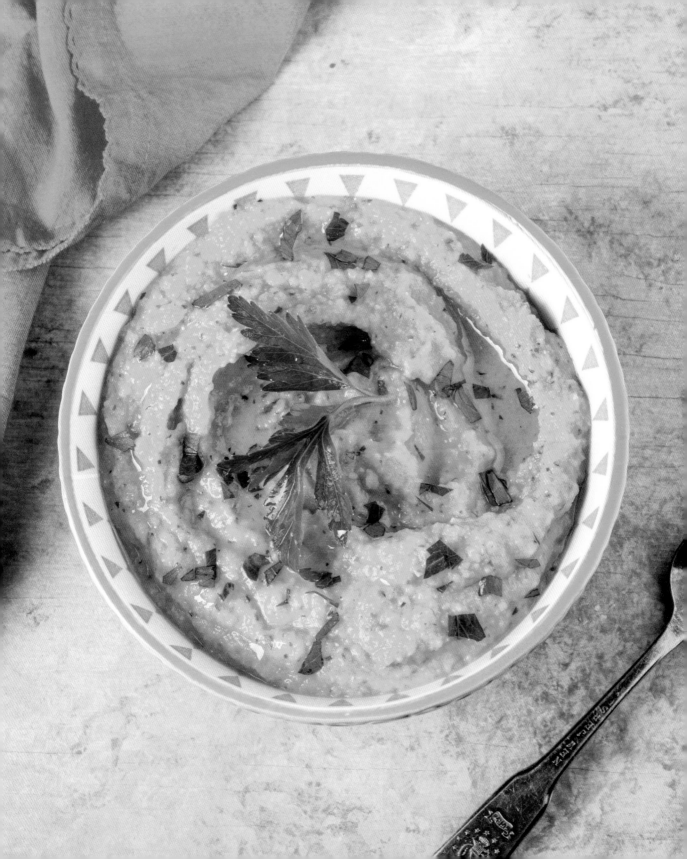

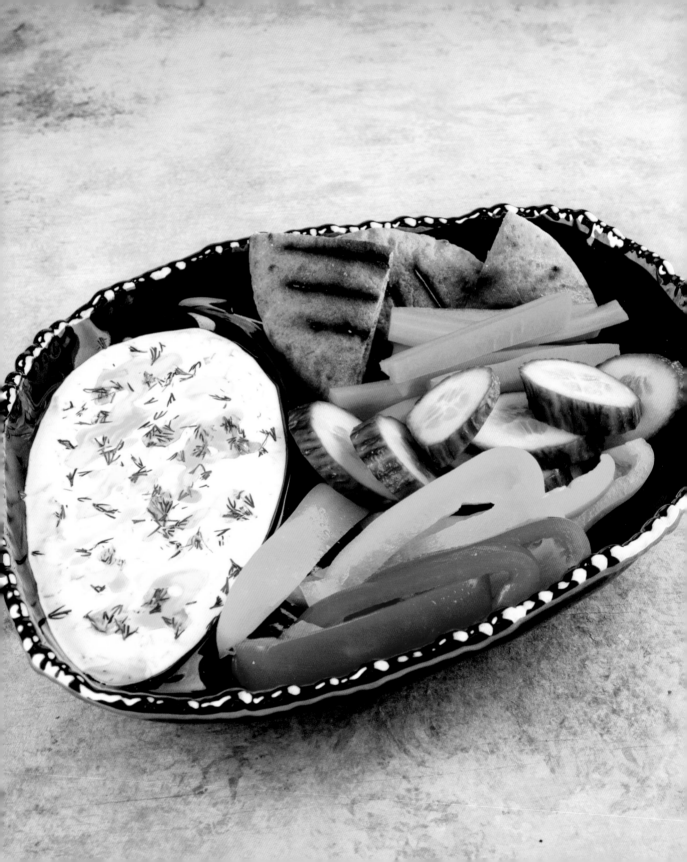

Refreshing Tzatziki

Tzatziki is a "must have" appetizer during any of my family's gatherings and many weeknight meals as well. Store-bought tzatziki can never taste as good as my mom's and there is no way that it is as healthy as hers. We prefer to dice the cucumber for a nice crunch, but it can also be grated. The lemon, cucumber and dill make this recipe so refreshing. It can be stored in the fridge for up to 4 days. Tzatziki is great accompanied by small bites such as Greek Meatballs (page 106).

Makes 6 servings

1½ cups (360 ml) plain Greek yogurt

2 Persian cucumbers, finely diced

2 cloves garlic, minced

3 tbsp (10 g) finely chopped fresh dill

1 tbsp (15 ml) fresh lemon juice

1 tbsp (15 ml) extra virgin olive oil, plus more for garnish

Sea salt to taste

Sliced cucumbers, for serving, optional

Sliced carrots, for serving, optional

Toasted pita, for serving, optional

In a large bowl, combine the Greek yogurt, cucumbers, garlic, dill, lemon juice, olive oil and salt. Mix well and transfer to a serving bowl. Drizzle with a tiny bit of olive oil to give it a beautiful gloss and chill for at least an hour in the fridge before serving.

Serve with sliced cucumbers, carrots and toasted pita if you desire or have it on its own.

Nedi's Tip: *To make this recipe vegan, replace the Greek yogurt with unsweetened coconut yogurt.*

Roasted Red Pepper Hummus

I absolutely love making hummus, but sometimes regular hummus can taste a bit bland, and that is why I love adding roasted red peppers to my hummus. They enhance the flavor and add extra vitamins and nutrients. Red peppers contain more than 200 percent of your daily vitamin C intake. The vitamin A and beta carotene in red peppers support eye health and overall vision. They are also delicious!

Makes 4 servings

1 (15-oz [425-g]) can chickpeas, rinsed and drained

2 roasted red peppers

2 cloves garlic

¼ cup (60 ml) tahini

2 tbsp (30 ml) extra virgin olive oil, plus more for drizzling

3 tbsp (45 ml) freshly squeezed lemon juice

1 jalapeño, seeds removed

1 tsp cumin

1 tsp sea salt

¼ tsp paprika

1 tbsp (4 g) chopped fresh parsley

Vegetable crudités, for serving, optional

Toasted pita, for serving, optional

Place the chickpeas, roasted red peppers, garlic, tahini, olive oil, lemon juice, jalapeño, cumin and salt in a food processor. Pulse until the mixture becomes smooth.

Transfer to a serving bowl. Drizzle with some olive oil, sprinkle with the paprika and garnish with the fresh parsley. Serve with vegetable crudités or toasted pita if you desire.

Nedi's Tip: *Try making this hummus with roasted green peppers and roasting the jalapeño. That will add a bit of smokiness to the dish and it's delicious.*

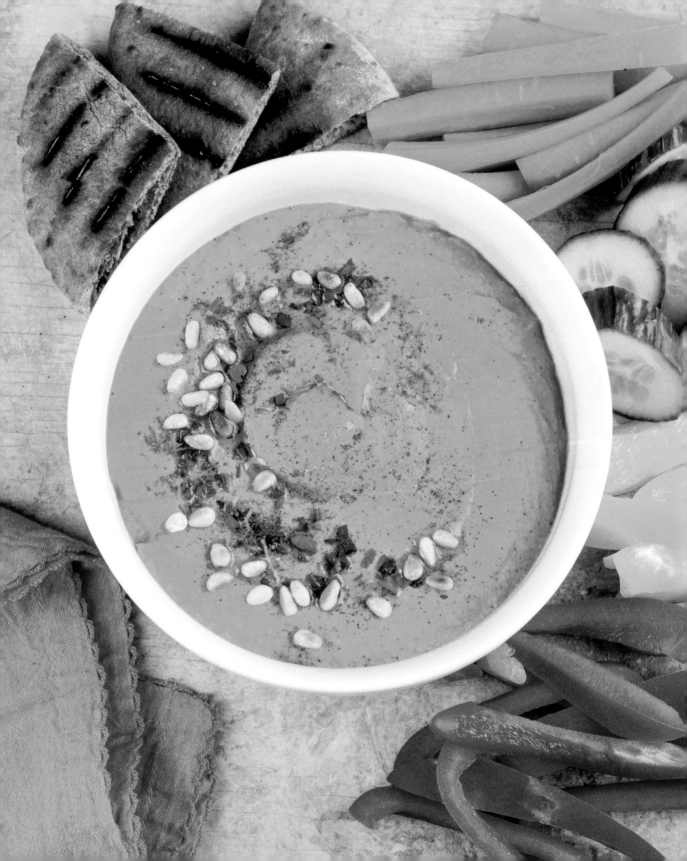

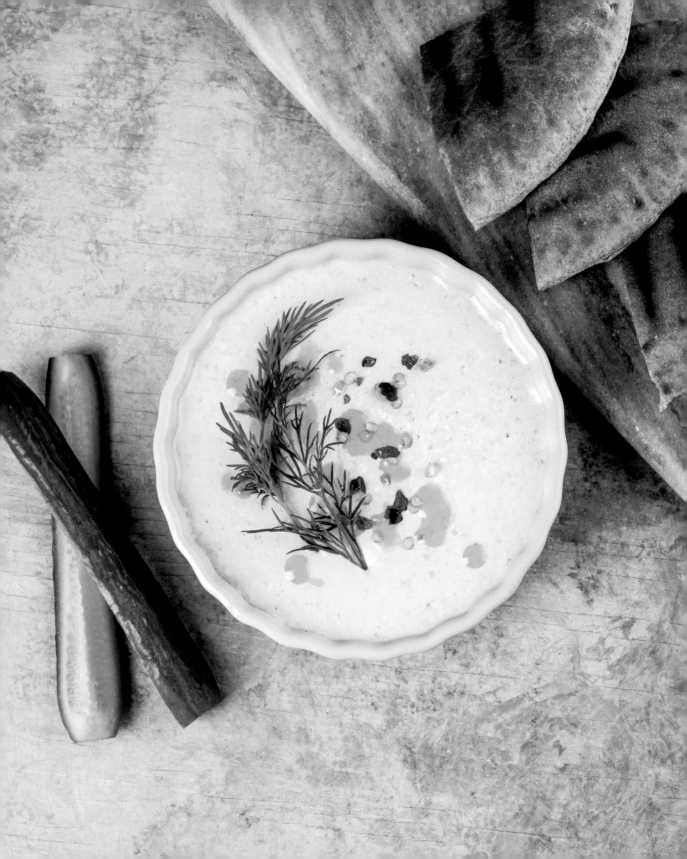

Spicy Greek Feta Dip (Tirokafteri)

Spice things up with this tangy and creamy dip! Tirokafteri in Greek means spicy cheese, so don't be afraid to use all the peppers. Remember that the yogurt and feta will somewhat neutralize the spicy taste, so if you like it very spicy, add one or two more peppers.

Makes 6 servings

1 clove garlic, sliced

3 Serrano peppers or jalapeños, seeds removed and chopped

2 tbsp (30 ml) plain Greek yogurt

12 oz (340 g) crumbled feta cheese

2 tbsp (30 ml) extra virgin olive oil, plus more for drizzling

1 tbsp (15 ml) fresh lemon juice or white wine vinegar

¼ tsp hot paprika

1 tbsp (3 g) finely chopped chives

Lemon slices, for serving, optional

Cucumber slices, for serving, optional

Place the garlic, Serrano peppers, Greek yogurt, feta, olive oil and fresh lemon juice in a food processor. Pulse for 20 to 30 seconds, until the mixture is well blended.

Transfer to a serving bowl and garnish with the hot paprika, a drizzle of olive oil and the chopped chives. Serve garnished with lemon and cucumber slices if desired.

Nedi's Tip: I've always loved eating this dip with keftedes, also known as Greek Meatballs (page 106), so give it a try and enjoy!

Creamy Baba Ganoush

Baba ganoush, also known as eggplant dip, is similar to hummus but uses eggplant instead of chickpeas. It's smoky, savory and super refreshing. I love all the Mediterranean flavors this dish packs. It is usually made with eggplant, tahini, olive oil and lemon. I personally love to add fresh parsley and a touch of cumin to take the flavors to the next level. I like to serve the baba ganoush with sliced vegetables, toasted pita or grilled meat.

Makes 4 servings

2 medium eggplants

3 cloves garlic, sliced

2 tbsp (8 g) fresh parsley, plus more for garnish

2 tbsp (30 ml) extra virgin olive oil

2 tbsp (30 ml) tahini

2 tbsp (30 ml) freshly squeezed lemon juice

¼ tsp cumin

Sea salt to taste

2 tbsp (25 g) pomegranate seeds

½ tsp paprika

Cherry tomatoes, for garnish, optional

Toasted pita, for garnish, optional

Preheat the oven to 450°F (230°C).

Line a baking dish with parchment paper. Halve the eggplants lengthwise and spray with olive oil cooking spray. Place them with the halved sides down and bake for 35 to 40 minutes. Set the eggplant aside to cool then scoop out the flesh with a spoon, leaving the skin behind.

Place the eggplant flesh in a food process and add the garlic, parsley, olive oil, tahini, lemon juice, cumin and salt. Pulse until smooth.

Transfer to a serving plate and garnish with the pomegranate seeds, paprika and fresh parsley. Enjoy it with cherry tomatoes and toasted pita if you like.

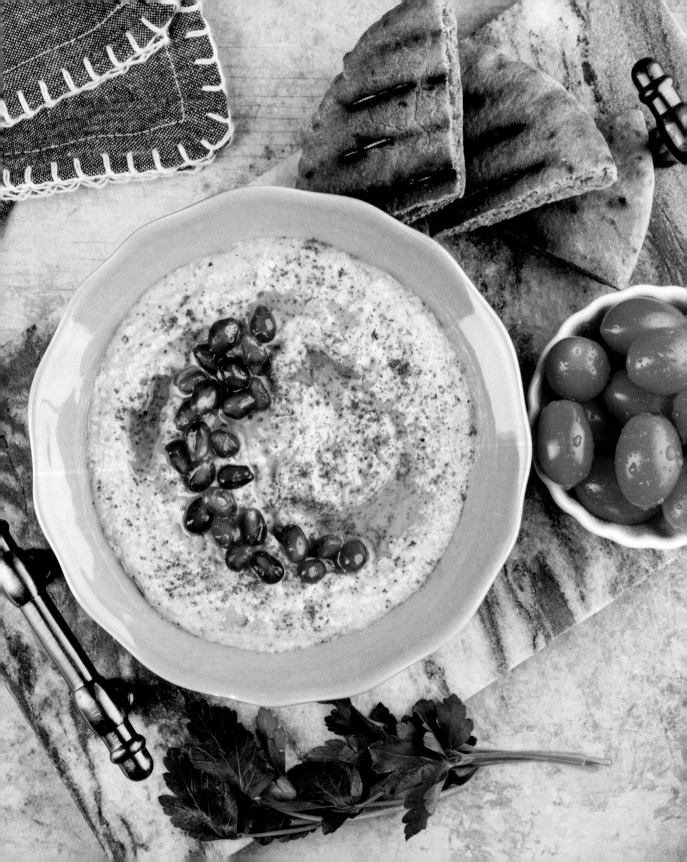

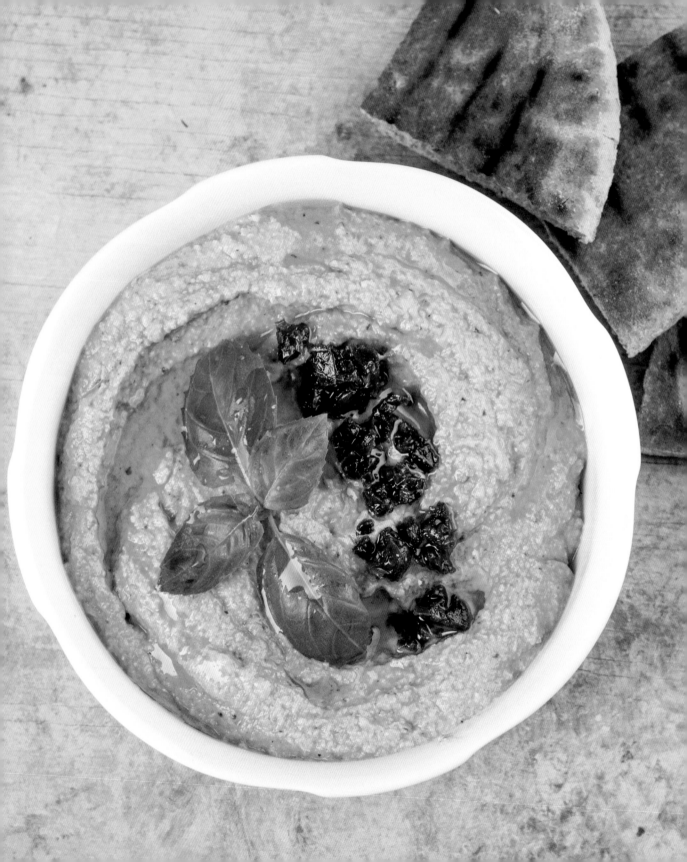

Fresh Artichoke Dip

This creamy dip is loaded with so many wonderful flavors. It will awaken your senses and will easily become one of your weekly staples. I love making fresh dips and having them available in my fridge during the week. They make a healthy snack and a great addition to wraps, sandwiches or grilled meats.

Makes 4 servings

1 (11-oz [312-g]) jar artichokes, drain and rinsed

1 tbsp (2 g) fresh basil, plus more for garnish

2 cloves garlic

2 tbsp (30 ml) plain Greek yogurt

2 tbsp (30 ml) extra virgin olive oil, plus more for drizzling

2 tbsp (10 g) grated pecorino Romano

1 tbsp (6 g) sun-dried tomatoes

1 tbsp (15 ml) freshly squeezed lemon juice

Sea salt and pepper to taste

Vegetable crudités, for serving

Toasted pita or sourdough bread, for serving

Place the artichokes, basil, garlic, Greek yogurt, olive oil, pecorino Romano, sun-dried tomatoes, lemon juice, salt and pepper in a food processor. Blend for 30 seconds, until smooth.

Transfer to a serving bowl. Drizzle with olive oil and garnish with fresh basil. Enjoy it with beautiful vegetable crudités spread and toasted pita or sourdough bread.

> Nedi's Tip: *Try adding a cup of fresh baby spinach to this dip. The combination of spinach and artichokes is delicious.*

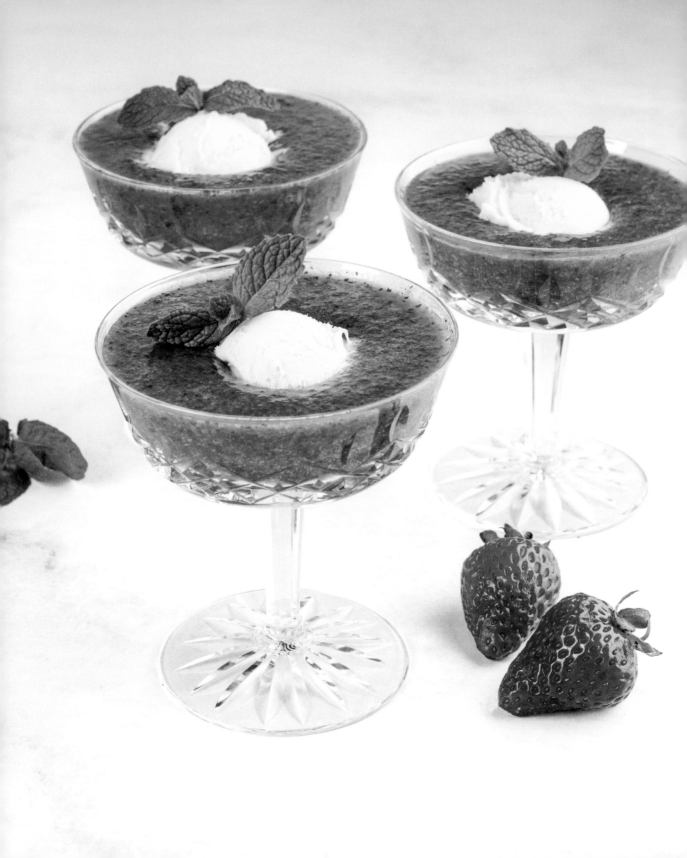

Mouthwatering Healthy Desserts

These Mediterranean-inspired desserts are made with fewer calories, carbohydrates and sugar than most desserts, but still taste luxurious and decadent. My "Healthy with Nedi"–approved dessert recipes include items such as Greek Baklava (page 157) and Greek Christmas Honey Cookies (page 165). I don't personally eat dessert every day, but when the sweet tooth kicks in or we have a special occasion, these stunning desserts are more than okay to be enjoyed in moderation.

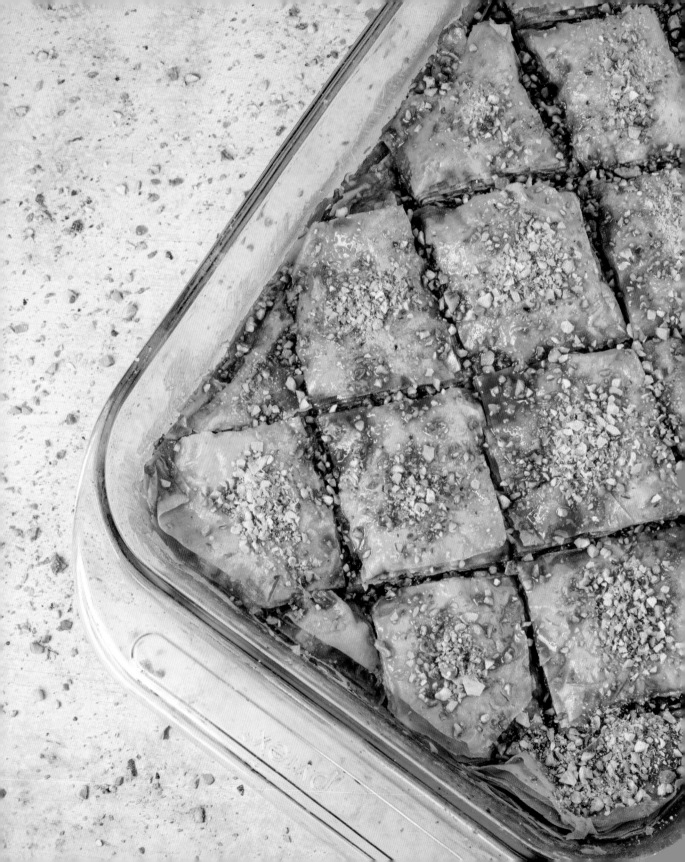

Greek Baklava

This Greek baklava is so easy to make, and everyone will think you are ready to win the next MasterChef after tasting it! To make this baklava perfect, make sure the sauce is completely cooled before pouring it over the hot baklava. Alternatively, the baklava can be prepared the day before and the sauce may be poured over the cooled baklava while the sauce is hot. Both ways work, but those steps are super important.

We like to serve this on holidays, and our Christmas dinner table always has baklava. Phyllo dough can be found in the freezer section of most grocery stores. The dough can be thawed in the fridge overnight or defrosted on the kitchen counter for a few hours.

Makes 10 servings

Baklava

2 cups (240 g) raw walnuts

3 tbsp (36 g) coconut sugar

1 tbsp (8 g) cinnamon

½ cup (1 stick/114 g) butter, melted

8 oz (226 g) thin phyllo dough sheets, thawed

2 tbsp (15 g) ground pistachios, for garnish

Syrup

1 cup (240 ml) water

⅔ cups (125 g) coconut sugar

½ cup (120 ml) honey

¼ cup (60 ml) fresh lemon juice

2 tbsp (30 ml) fresh orange juice

1 tsp vanilla extract

Preheat the oven to 375°F (190°C). Grease the bottom and sides of a 9 x 13–inch (20 x 23–cm) pan with cooking spray.

Finely chop the walnuts with a knife or in a food processor. In a bowl, toss the nuts with the coconut sugar and cinnamon. Set aside.

Place one sheet of dough in the pan, then generously coat with melted butter using a silicone brush. Add another sheet of dough and brush again with the melted butter. Repeat until you have eight sheets layered. Sprinkle half of the nut mixture on top.

Add another five sheets of buttered phyllo dough, then top with the remaining nut mixture. Finish the final layers with eight sheets of buttered phyllo dough.

Cut the pastry into wide strips lengthwise, then cut diagonally to form diamond shapes. Bake for 25 to 30 minutes, until golden brown. Remove the pan from the oven and set it aside to cool completely for a few hours.

Meanwhile, prepare the syrup. In a small pot, bring the water to a boil and add the coconut sugar, honey, lemon juice, orange juice and vanilla. Lower the heat and simmer for 20 minutes. Let the syrup rest for 2 to 3 minutes to cool slightly.

Pour the hot syrup over the completely cooled baklava. Garnish with the ground pistachios and set aside for a few hours so the baklava can absorb the syrup.

The baklava can be stored at room temperature for up to 2 weeks.

> Nedi's Tip: *Try making this baklava with 1 cup (120 g) of walnuts and 1 cup (120 g) of pistachios or hazelnuts. Sometimes I like to combine the nuts, and the flavors are impeccable.*

Hazelnut Cookies with Orange Zest

These hazelnut cookies are unbelievably delicious. Imagine the combination of something that tastes like Nutella with coconut and a hint of orange . . . only much healthier, vegan and gluten-free! These cookies are easy to make and can last in the fridge for a week. Although, that is never the case in my house because they are gone within a day!

Try to purchase roasted and peeled hazelnuts to save time. If they aren't already roasted, roast them for 10 minutes at 350°F (175°C) to enhance the flavor and make sure to remove the peels.

Makes 13 cookies

2 cups (270 g) roasted peeled hazelnuts

1 tbsp (15 ml) coconut oil

2 tbsp (22 g) coconut flour

Pinch of sea salt

2 tbsp (30 ml) maple syrup

Zest of ½ orange

1 oz (28 g) dark chocolate

Add the hazelnuts to a food processor with the coconut oil and pulse for 2 to 3 minutes, until a creamy hazelnut butter consistency forms. Add the coconut flour, salt, maple syrup and the orange zest. Pulse until well combined.

Line a large plate with parchment paper and form egg-shaped cookies. This recipe will make approximately 13 small, egg-shaped cookies. Place the plate in the freezer for 20 minutes.

Melt the dark chocolate in a small bowl in the microwave for 30 seconds (or longer if needed) then dip the cookies in chocolate so that only half of the cookie is covered. Place the cookies in the refrigerator for 1 hour and take them out 5 minutes before ready to eat. (If they stay out at room temperature for too long, they may start to soften and melt.)

Nedi's Tip: *To lower the sugar and carb content, try replacing the maple syrup with yacon syrup. Yacon syrup is extracted from the roots of the yacon plant. It is effective against constipation and may lower blood sugar levels.*

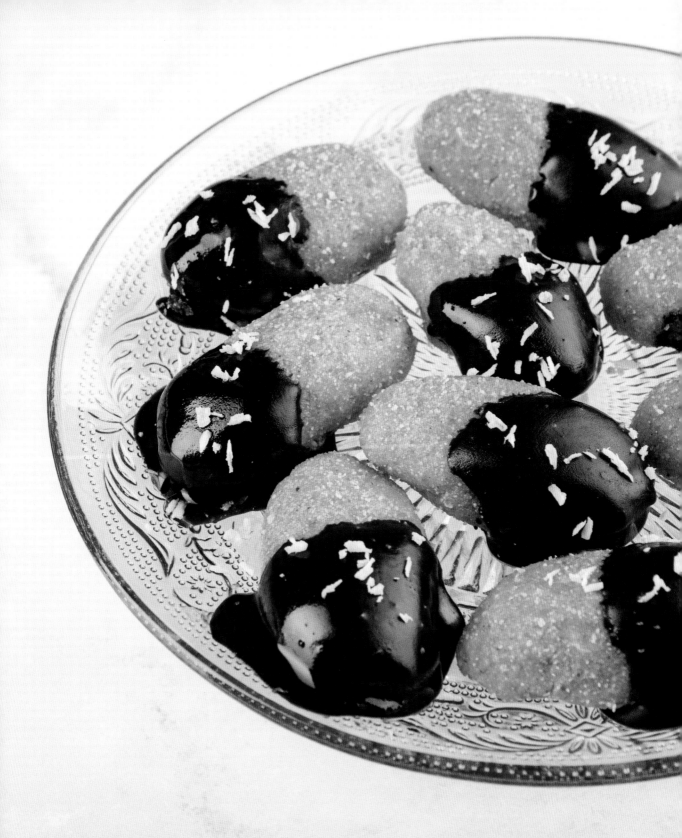

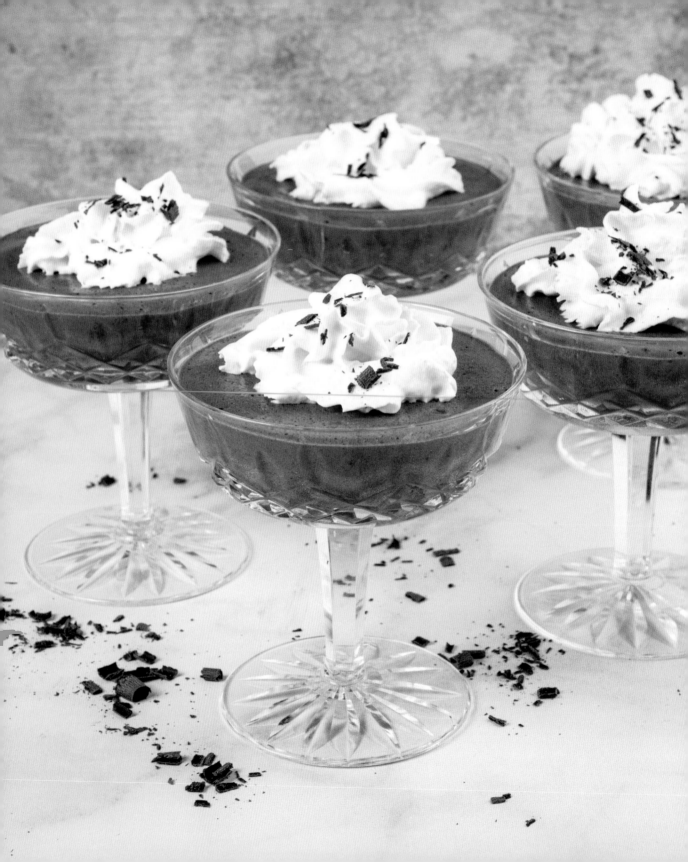

Light and Airy Chocolate Mousse

This chocolate mousse is airy and light, yet rich and flavorful with a silky-smooth texture. It makes a fancy dessert and will easily impress guests, yet you won't believe how easy it is to make. My mom and I had a lot of fun finalizing this recipe. We tested it several times and on the last trial we ran out of chocolate at 9 p.m. I remember rushing to the store as we had all the eggs separated and ready to be mixed in with the chocolate. This cookbook truly is a labor of love, and each recipe has a special memory to it. The late-night grocery run was totally worth it. This turned out to be the most decadent chocolate mousse I have ever tried.

Makes 6 servings

6 eggs

2 tsp (10 ml) lemon juice

Pinch of sea salt

1 tsp vanilla extract

7 oz (200 g) dark chocolate chips

2 tbsp (30 ml) coconut cream

Heavy whipping cream, whipped to soft peaks, for garnish, optional

Cacao powder or chocolate shavings, for garnish, optional

Separate the egg yolks from the whites and place the whites in a medium-sized bowl and the yolks in a separate medium-sized bowl.

To the egg white bowl, add the lemon juice and pinch of salt. Whisk with a hand mixer until stiff peaks form.

Add the vanilla to the egg yolk bowl and whisk with a hand mixer.

In a large heatproof bowl, heat the chocolate and coconut cream in the microwave in 30-second intervals, stirring in between each one, until the chocolate is melted and the mixture is smooth.

Let the mixture cool for a few minutes, then whisk in the egg yolks slowly, until smooth. Fold the egg whites into the chocolate and mix with a spatula.

Divide the mixture evenly among six dessert glasses, then cover and chill in the refrigerator until set, at least 2 hours. Take the glasses out of the fridge for 15 minutes before serving so the mousse can soften.

Serve topped with whipped cream and cacao powder or shavings, if desired.

> Nedi's Tip: This is a perfect dessert to serve during the holidays and it can be prepared a day or two ahead of the party.

Apple and Cinnamon Muffins

These muffins will quickly become one of your favorite treats. They are so tasty; plus, apples and cinnamon go together like peanut butter and jelly. The muffins are gluten and dairy-free, and packed with nutrients, fiber and protein. Cinnamon provides antibacterial and anti-inflammatory properties, curbs sugar cravings and lowers blood sugar levels.

These muffins are wonderful for breakfast with a cup of coffee and a teaspoon of nut butter.

Makes 9 servings

2 cups (190 g) almond meal/flour

½ cup (100 g) monkfruit sweetener or coconut sugar

2 tbsp (22 g) chia seeds

1½ tbsp (12 g) cinnamon

1 tsp baking powder

3 tbsp (45 ml) coconut or plain Greek yogurt

1 tsp baking soda

2 eggs

2 apples, grated and water squeezed out

2 tbsp (30 ml) coconut oil, melted

2 tbsp (30 ml) nut milk

Preheat the oven to 350°F (175°C). Line a muffin tin with muffin liners. Lightly spray each liner with coconut oil cooking spray.

In a large bowl, combine the almond meal/flour, monkfruit or coconut sugar, chia seeds, cinnamon and baking powder. Mix thoroughly.

In a small bowl, mix the yogurt with the baking soda and let it rise for a minute. Add the eggs and whisk well. Add this mixture to the dry ingredients. Add the grated apples, coconut oil and nut milk to the mixture. Mix using a fork, until well combined.

Pour the mixture into the muffin liners; it should be enough to fill nine muffin molds. Bake for 25 to 30 minutes, until golden.

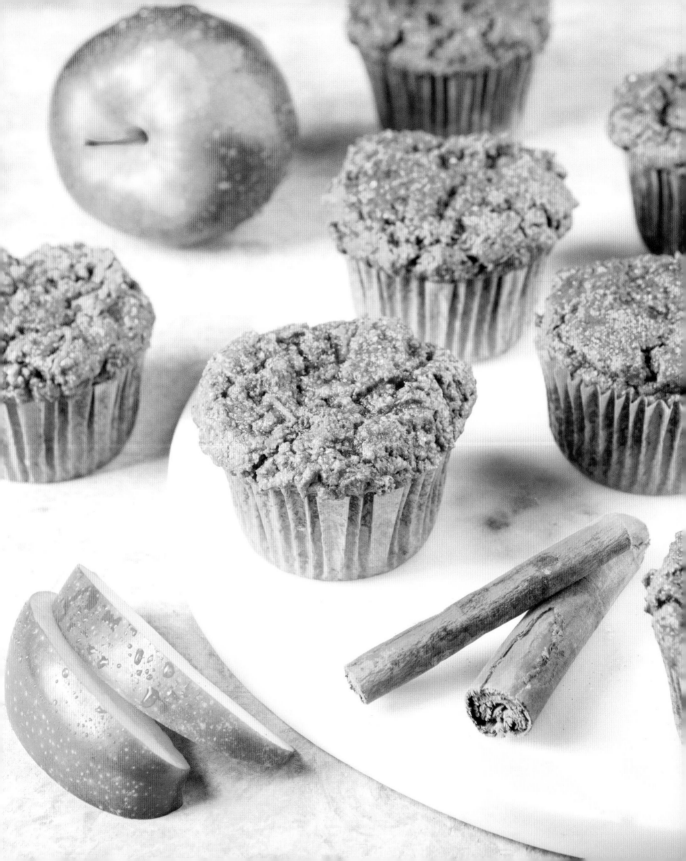

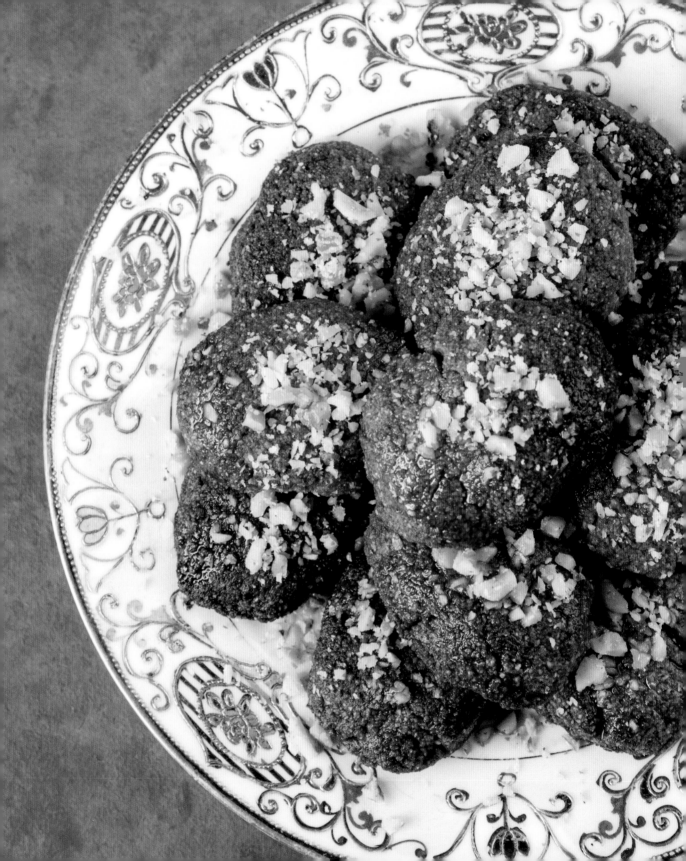

Greek Christmas Honey Cookies (Melomakarona)

These are traditional Greek cookies that are made during Christmas. While I usually don't have much of a sweet tooth, I seriously wait all year for them and can never get enough. They are soft and chewy with just the perfect amount of crunch. The flavors will make your taste buds go crazy. A combination of honey, cinnamon, and orange . . . sweet with a slight twist of zest.

Makes 30 cookies

¾ cup (180 ml) water

⅓ cup (65 g) coconut sugar

½ cup (120 ml) honey

1 cinnamon stick

½ orange

2 tbsp (30 ml) fresh lemon juiced

1 cup (240 ml) extra virgin olive oil

¼ cup (60 ml) fresh orange juice

Zest of 1 orange

2 tbsp (30 ml) honey

3 tbsp (45 ml) brandy

3½ cups (335 g) almond meal/flour

4 tbsp (44 g) coconut flour

1 tsp cinnamon

1 tsp baking powder

½ tsp baking soda

½ cup (60 g) walnuts, chopped, for garnish

In a medium saucepan, combine the water, coconut sugar, honey, cinnamon stick, orange half and the lemon juice. Bring to a boil then lower the heat to medium. Cook for 5 minutes and set the syrup aside to cool. It's important to let the syrup cool completely so the fresh warm cookies can better absorb it. The sauce can be prepared a day ahead or in the morning of the day you plan to make the cookies.

Preheat the oven to 350°F (175°C). Line a baking sheet with parchment paper.

In a large bowl, combine the olive oil, orange juice, orange zest, honey and brandy. Mix well.

In a medium bowl, sift the almond meal/flour, coconut flour, cinnamon, baking powder and baking soda. Mix, then add to the large bowl with the liquid batter. Mix until the ingredients are well combined.

Form 30 oval cookies, about 1 tablespoon (15 g) each, using a spoon or cookie scoop. Place them on the parchment-lined baking sheet. Lightly press the center of each cookie down with a fork to flatten a bit (don't push too hard because you don't want the cookies completely flat). Bake the cookies for 20 to 25 minutes, until brown. Allow the cookies to cool slightly.

Remove the orange and cinnamon stick from the cooled syrup. Dip each warm cookie into the syrup for 15 to 20 seconds. Do this in batches, making sure all the cookies absorb enough syrup. Using a slotted spoon, remove the cookies from the syrup and place them on a serving dish. Sprinkle the cookies with the chopped walnuts and enjoy!

> **Nedi's Tips:** *It is very important that the syrup is completely cool so the warm cookies can soak it up.*
>
> *Make sure you don't soak each cookie for longer than 15 to 20 seconds because they will become too soft and may break.*

Flourless Chocolate Cake with Walnuts

This is the most delicious, decadent, flourless chocolate cake that you will ever taste. My mom used to make this cake for birthdays and special family gatherings all the time. We have made the perfect tweaks to make sure it can be enjoyed in this Mediterranean meal guide. The ingredients consist mainly of chocolate, walnuts, eggs, butter and coconut oil. After all, there is no better combination than chocolate and coconut. Chocolate lovers will love this dessert!

Makes 8 servings

6 eggs, at room temperature

Pinch of sea salt

½ tsp fresh lemon juice

1 ½ cups (180 g) walnuts, finely chopped

½ cup (1 stick/114 g) soft butter, plus more to grease the pan

¼ cup (60 ml) coconut oil

½ cup (96 g) coconut sugar

2 tbsp (30 ml) honey

2 tbsp (10 g) cacao powder

1 oz (50 g) dark chocolate

Sliced strawberries, for serving, optional

Preheat the oven to 350°F (175°C). Grease an 8-inch (20-cm) cake pan with butter and place a piece of parchment paper on the bottom. Cut the paper to fit exactly in the pan.

Separate the yolks from the egg whites and place each in separate bowls.

In a large mixing bowl, beat the egg whites with a pinch of salt and the lemon juice using a mixer until they become white and fluffy, about 2 minutes. Add the walnuts to the bowl with the egg whites.

In a smaller bowl, beat the soft butter, coconut oil, coconut sugar and honey with a mixer. Add the egg yolks and cacao powder and beat until mixed well.

Take half of the mixture from the egg yolk bowl and add it to the bowl of egg whites and walnuts. Set aside the other half of the egg yolk mixture.

Add the egg white mixture to the prepared pan and bake for 15 to 20 minutes. Insert a toothpick in the cake; if it comes out with no crumbs, the cake is ready.

Let the cake cool completely then transfer to a serving platter. When completely cool, spread the remaining egg yolk mixture on top and over the sides. Grate the dark chocolate on top and serve with sliced strawberries if you like.

> Nedi's Tip: *If the walnuts are not already chopped, then add them into a small food processor and pulse until they become finely chopped.*

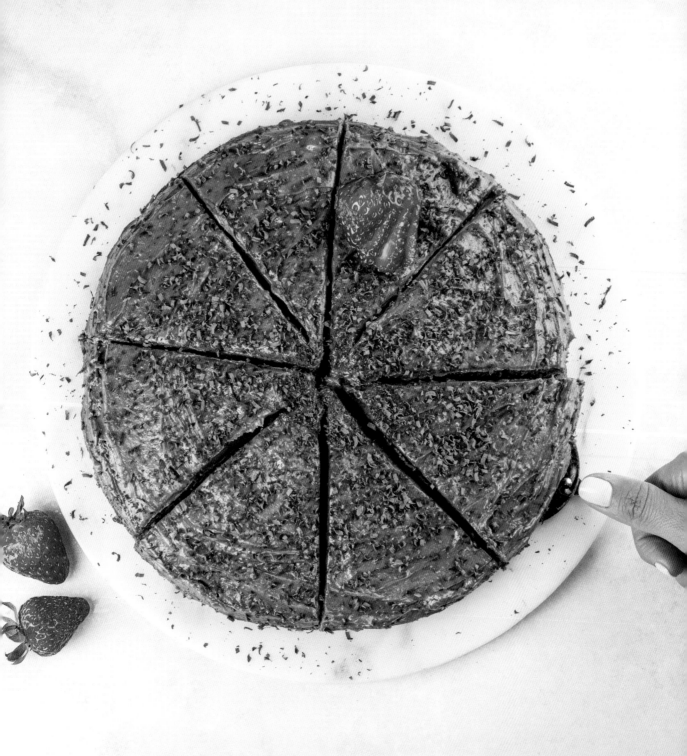

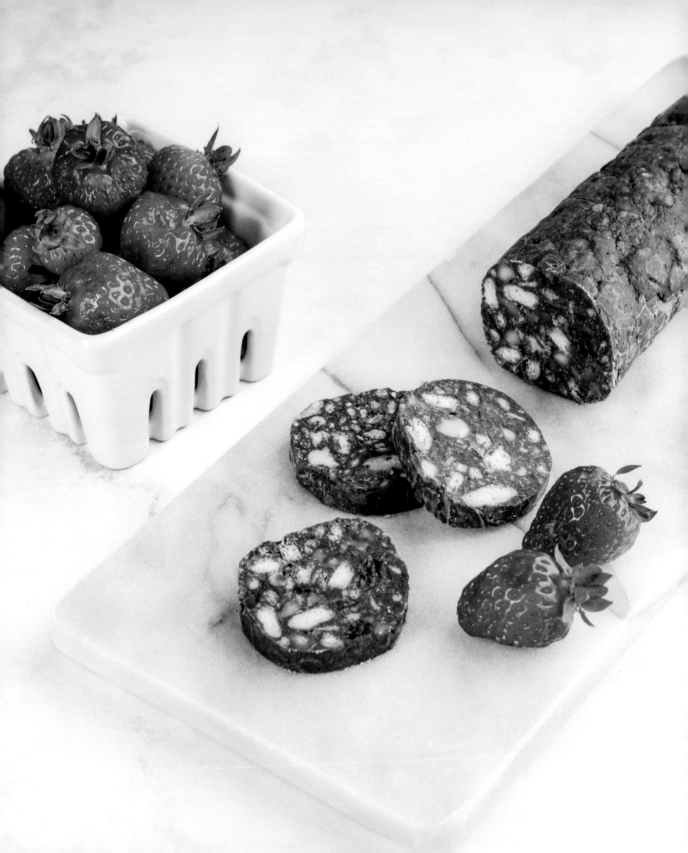

Raw Chocolate Salami

This chocolate salami is an old family recipe that my mom and yiayia always used to make when I was a child. It brings back many of my favorite childhood memories and I am so happy to share this recipe with you. The chocolate salami can be made in many different ways using different gluten-free cookies/biscuits as a base and your choice of nuts and dried fruit. I find that raisins and dates work best for this recipe, but you can get creative and try out another dried fruit like figs or prunes. This is a fast and easy, no-bake dessert that can be premade and stored in the fridge.

Makes 8 servings

1½ cups (168 g) crumbled cinnamon cookies (I used Simple Mill's Snickerdoodle cookies)

1 cup (120 g) walnuts, chopped

3 tbsp (30 g) dates, chopped

1 tbsp (5 g) cocoa powder

3.5 oz (100 g) dark chocolate, melted

3 tbsp (45 ml) coconut oil, melted

3 tbsp (45 ml) coconut milk

1 tsp vanilla extract

1 tbsp (15 ml) amaretto

Sliced strawberries, for garnish, optional

In a bowl, combine the cookie crumbs, walnuts, dates and cocoa powder. Mix well and set aside.

In a separate bowl, combine the melted chocolate, melted coconut oil, coconut milk, vanilla and amaretto. Mix then add the dry mixture. Stir until well combined.

Place the mixture on a large piece of parchment paper and roll into a log shape. Wrap it with the parchment paper and place it in the fridge for 2 to 3 hours, or overnight. Take the salami out of the fridge 5 minutes before you are ready to serve, then slice and garnish with the sliced strawberries if using.

Nedi's Tips: To create the cookie crumbles, place the cookies in a zip-lock bag and lightly crush them into small pieces with a rolling pin or similar object, then measure.

I like to prepare two or three salamis at once and store them in the freezer. They can stay fresh for up to 3 months and make an impressive last-minute dessert.

Sweet Strawberry Gazpacho

This refreshing dessert is not just tasty but is also loaded with nutrients. It doesn't require a lot of time in the kitchen, and the flavors and color are perfect for summer. This strawberry gazpacho will easily become your favorite summer dessert.

Makes 4 servings

¼ cup (60 ml) lukewarm water

2 tbsp (24 g) coconut sugar

1 lb (454 g) strawberries

Juice of 1 lime

¼ cup (23 g) fresh mint leaves, reserve four leaves for garnish

2 tbsp (3 g) fresh basil

4 small scoops dairy-free vanilla ice cream

In a small bowl, mix the warm water with the coconut sugar until it melts. Add the sugar water mixture to a food processor and add the strawberries, lime juice, mint and basil leaves. Blend until well combined.

Pour the strawberry mixture into four small dessert glasses or bowls. Chill in the fridge for a few hours before serving. Serve with a scoop of dairy-free vanilla ice cream and a mint leaf.

Nedi's Tip: *This dessert can be stored in the fridge for up to 3 days.*

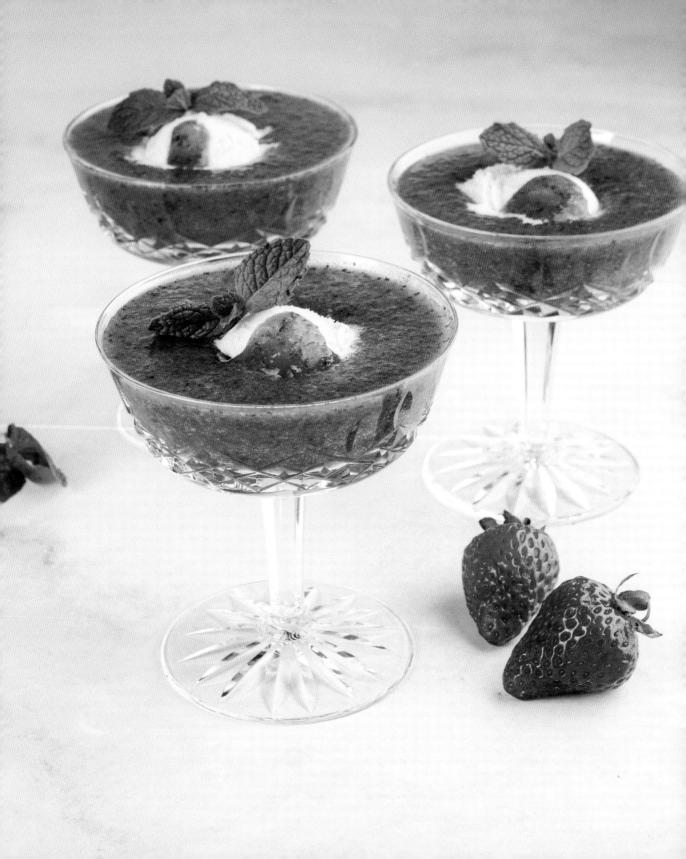

Acknowledgments

First and foremost, I'd like to say thank you to anyone who has read and followed Healthy with Nedi. Thank you for your ongoing support and being on this journey with me.

Mom—You have been my biggest supporter since day one. I owe so much to you and I'm grateful for everything you have taught me. Spending time in the kitchen with you is one of my all-time favorite things to do. We have cooked so many recipes and have created unforgettable memories. Thank you so much for helping me test the recipes in this book and being my number one recipe tester! I love you so much.

Yiayia—I am so lucky to have you in my life. Our bond is so special that my best friends always joke and say they want to find someone who loves them as much as I love you! You have always pushed me to chase after my dreams. Your warm advice is golden, and I will treasure your wise words forever. You have hand-written many notebooks with recipes, guidance and health tips, and I'm so happy I can apply parts of them in this cookbook.

Vuicho—In loving memory of my uncle. Even though you were not the healthiest eater, you loved when I experimented with new recipes and were always excited to try a healthier version of your favorite meals. I know how much our family meals meant to you and I will cherish those times forever in my heart.

Dan—You are the best stepdad a daughter could ever dream of. It means so much to me that you are always eager to try out my recipe modifications and what makes me smile the most is when you don't notice the substitutes I make! Your honest opinion and feedback have been so helpful.

Jacqui Somen—You have been by my side since the very early days of Healthy with Nedi. You believed in me from the get-go! Thank you for making my work with you so enjoyable.

Debbie Puig—I have no words to express my gratitude for your help with the recipe testing along the way. I admire your love and passion for health and cooking.

Oksana Fedali—Thank you for the most stunning images and making my recipes look so delicious. We are the dream team, and I am so grateful for our friendship.

Page Street Publishing and my editor Sarah Monroe—I am beyond grateful for your hard work as we brought this cookbook to life. You helped me make this huge dream into reality.

Vani Hari—Thank you for your guidance and being a huge mentor to me. Your endless research, love and devotion to health and making the world a better place is truly inspiring. I have such admiration for you, both personally and professionally.

Nikki Sharp and Maria Marlowe—Thank you for all of your help during the writing of my cookbook proposal. I appreciate you sharing your own personal experiences with me.

To all my best friends who came over and taste-tested almost every recipe, thank you for always giving me your honest opinion, for believing in me and my message.

About The Author

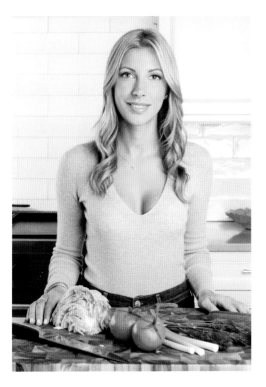

Neda Varbanova is the creator of Healthy with Nedi, a website designed to share innovative healthy recipes and lifestyle tips. Neda's culinary creations are centered around fresh foods and are inspired by her time in the kitchen with her beloved mother and grandmother in Bulgaria and Greece.

When Neda first arrived in the United States during middle school, she found that the American diet left her feeling ill. She quickly returned to her roots and began eating a Mediterranean-inspired diet again. This shift restored her health and reinvigorated her. Neda's experience motivated her to dedicate her life to sharing the pleasures of eating wholesome, fresh, Mediterranean-inspired meals with everyone she meets.

Neda's journey has led her to continually increase her knowledge about healthy food. She holds a master's in food studies from New York University Steinhardt, a certificate in culinary nutrition from the Natural Gourmet Institute and is a certified health coach through the Institute for Integrative Nutrition. Her work has been featured in *Elle*, *Grazia*, The Chalkboard, Well + Good, Healthline, mindbodygreen, Greatist, *Business Insider*, NBC News and more. You can find Neda at www.HealthyWithNedi.com and on social media @HealthyWithNedi.

Index